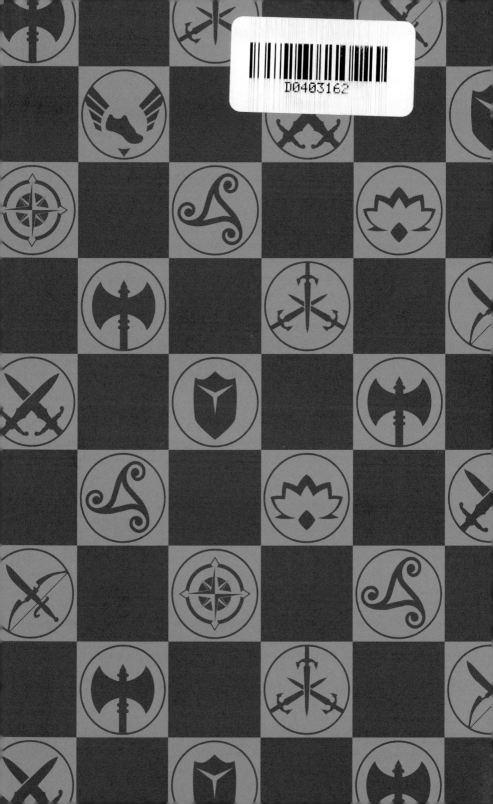

LEVEL UP YOUR LIFE

LEVEL UP YOUR LIFE

HOW TO UNLOCK ADVENTURE AND HAPPINESS
BY BECOMING THE HERO OF YOUR OWN STORY

STEVE KAMB
FOUNDER OF NERDFITNESS.COM

RODALE.

RODALE *wellness*

Live happy. Be healthy. Get inspired.

Sign up today to get exclusive access to our authors, exclusive bonuses, and the most authoritative, useful, and cutting edge information on health, wellness, fitness, and living your life to the fullest.

Visit us online at RodaleWellness.com
Join us at RodaleWellness.com/Join

Copyright © 2016 by Stephen Kamb

All rights reserved. No part of this publication may be reproduced or transmitted in any form or by any means, electronic or mechanical, including photocopying, recording, or any other information storage and retrieval system, without the written permission of the publisher.

Rodale books may be purchased for business or promotional use or for special sales. For information, please write to: Special Markets Department, Rodale, Inc., 733 Third Avenue, New York, NY 10017.

Printed in the United States of America

Rodale Inc. makes every effort to use acid-free ∞, recycled paper ♻.

Book design by Joanna Williams

Rebel Icons and chart on page 140 by Darryl Jones

Word balloons by Getty Images

Library of Congress Cataloging-in-Publication Data is on file with the publisher.

ISBN 978-1-62336-540-0   hardcover

Distributed to the trade by Macmillan.

2   4   6   8   10   9   7   5   3   1   hardcover

We inspire and enable people to improve their lives and the world around them.
rodalebooks.com

DEDICATION

FOR MY PARENTS, BROTHER, AND SISTER, WHO HAVE BEEN MY MOST SUPPORTIVE FANS SINCE DAY ONE—THANKS FOR TELLING ME TO GO FOR IT ANY TIME I BROUGHT UP A RIDICULOUS IDEA. MOM, I PROMISE I'LL CONTINUE TO TELL YOU ABOUT THE CRAZY THINGS ONLY AFTER I'VE ALREADY DONE THEM.

FOR MY GRANDMOTHER, WHO READS MY NEWSLETTERS, EVEN THOUGH SHE DOESN'T UNDERSTAND A LOT OF THEM—THANKS FOR PUTTING UP WITH MY FOUL LANGUAGE, GRAMMA! FOR MY OTHER GRANDPARENTS WHO, AFTER LIVING LONG INSPIRING LIVES, PASSED AWAY WHILE I WAS ON MY ADVENTURES. I MISS YOU GUYS.

FOR THE REBELLION! THANKS TO THE NERD FITNESS COMMUNITY, FULL OF UNLIKELY HEROES AND GOOFBALLS, FOR PUTTING MY WORDS INTO ACTION AND LIVING A LIFE FULL OF ADVENTURE EVERY DAY.

FOR THE CRAZY ONES. THE MISFITS. THE REBELS. THE TROUBLEMAKERS. THE ROUND PEGS IN THE SQUARE HOLES. THE ONES WHO SEE THINGS DIFFERENTLY.

CONTENTS

LEVELING UP—ADVANCE IN THE GAME OF LIFE

MASTERING ORDEALS—ACTIVATE BEAST MODE

THE ROAD BACK—CONTINUE? OR GAME OVER?

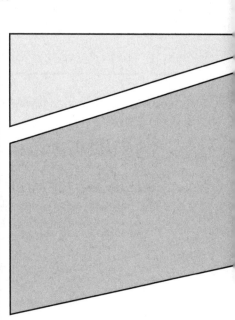

INTRODUCTION:
THE ORDINARY WORLD

BOND. JAMES BOND.   *—SEAN CONNERY, DR. NO*

Monte Carlo Casino, Monaco. 2 a.m.: "Hit me."

I sat at a blackjack table in the most famous casino in the world, and my heart started pounding. After splitting my hand three times and doubling down twice, I struggled to stay cool and calm under pressure; after all, although it wasn't a tremendous amount of money, I had nearly as much riding on that one hand of blackjack as I had spent in the entire previous week. I ordered another cocktail (shaken, not stirred), adjusted the bow tie on my tuxedo, and cracked a corny joke to my new friends from Ireland sitting next to me. The rest of the table played their hands, then the dealer slowly turned over his cards, hit, and busted. The table exploded with applause, and I calmly collected my chips while internally dancing a jig and freaking out.

After partying into the wee hours of the night with new friends, I returned to my hotel on the Mediterranean, literally—the Fairmont Monte Carlo is actually on stilts over the water. I awoke the next morning, enjoyed a breakfast watching billion-dollar yachts pulling into Monaco's harbor, and proudly crossed a massive item off my gamified bucket list, appropriately named Steve's "Epic

Quest of Awesome": Live like James Bond for a weekend.

I doubt anybody who had seen me that night in the casino would have believed who I really was and how my life had changed over the previous year. They probably weren't aware I had rented my tuxedo from an actual costume shop in the next town over, or that my hotel was paid for with hotel points and cost me nothing. Nor would they know that despite the lavish weekend, I was actually quite frugal and thanks to my run of luck at the tables I had managed to make money on the weekend! Lastly, who would expect that the witty (hopefully) charming gentleman in the tux gambling at the Monte Carlo would return the next day to a cheap hostel in Nice and return to life as a risk-averse, shy nerd?

How I lived out this double-life would surprise anybody, especially considering my starting point. Like many young people growing up in the 1980s, I spent most of my life occupied with my favorite books, video games, and movies for one key reason: escape. Escape from another day at school in which I wasn't challenged, wasn't captivated, and didn't grow. Escape from another day at a job in which I wasn't engaged, stuck in a position that didn't line up with my strengths. Escape from another day in life that wasn't nearly as interesting as the lives lived by the heroic characters in the games I played.

Why bother spending time in the real world, where I had to deal with things that made me miserable, where I was unhealthy, unhappy, uninspired, and where there wasn't any real excitement? Why bother with any of that when I could simply hop on my computer or game console and live out my fantasies as an epic, all-powerful badass capable of world domination? In real life I was a skinny twenty-something with no savings, no true direction, and mounting social anxiety. In a game world though, I could slay freaking dragons. It wasn't long before real life became the boring parts between the hours I spent plugging myself into adventures on the screen.

After all, it's fun to get lost in a book or a movie, or to jump into a video game world where you get to be the hero. I imagined myself as Indiana Jones, Jason Bourne, Neo from *The Matrix*, and even Link from the classic Nintendo game series, The Legend of Zelda. And there's nothing inherently wrong with any of that. I still love those games and movies and enjoy the entertainment they provide. They're a part of who I am as a person. The problem was that they had become a way to avoid the unhappiness in my real life while also allowing me to continue doing nothing about it.

And one day, something changed. Instead of losing myself in games and using them to escape, I put the wheels in motion to start doing all the amazing things I used to dream of. I turned my life into a giant video game, and lived out the fantasies of the characters I adored.

When I was 25, I had never once traveled outside of North America; since then, I've traveled to more than 20 countries, hiked the Great Wall of China, tracked wild animals in South Africa, explored the ruins of Angkor Wat in Cambodia, and gotten into the best shape of my life. When I'm not on an adventure, I volunteer my time regularly and play music every day. Most important, I'm happy.

And that's just a small part of what I've done. A friend and I hiked in the early morning hours up to a viewpoint overlooking the ancient ruins of Machu Picchu in Peru, which gave me the courage to take another big leap that resulted in a 2-year around-the-world adventure.

I woke up one morning on a bus in New Zealand and overheard the bus driver saying something about a "stunt plane." Less than 24 hours later I was completing barrel rolls and corkscrews in a stunt biplane (with the help of a copilot), living out my childhood fantasy of "keeping up foreign relations" just like Maverick did in the movie *Top Gun*.

A few days after flying an airplane, I jumped out of one. Two days after that? I jumped off Kawarau Bridge, birthplace of the bungee jump, and plunged myself waist-deep into an ice-cold river before shooting out of the water like a rocket into space.

There was that one night when I went scuba diving with sharks on the Great Barrier Reef. We sat on the boat preparing to dive, with rain pouring in sideways and AC/DC blasting over the boat's PA system, as large sharks circled the boat. I felt like I was living out a scene from a Tom Clancy novel. After surviving that adventure, I spent the next day exploring a vividly colored coral reef that housed a bright pink anemone and an adorable little clownfish. That's right: I found Nemo. Mission: complete!

In addition to my traveling adventures, I've found other ways to level up my life by implementing game mechanics into the rest of my life too. While writing this book, I also managed to pack on 15 pounds of muscle, learned to play the violin, dabbled with swing dance lessons, and volunteered every Thursday at a local children's hospital. It's been a rewarding, challenging, and fulfilling experience and I'm damn proud of it.

I'm not telling you all of this as someone who's been predestined for a life of adventure, or even to boast about how great my life has become. Quite the opposite, actually. Instead, I'm telling you all this as a risk-averse, picky-eating introvert who felt more at home in front of a computer than in public, and who has since become a world traveling adrenaline junkie. How did I do it? By hacking my source code and rewriting the expectations that others had for me (and the expectations I had for myself). By implementing cheat codes and shortcuts wherever possible to achieve results faster. By putting steps in place to move me a little bit closer each and every day from the life I lived to the life I wanted to live. I essentially reverse engineered my life around my Epic Quest of Awesome, systematically eliminating the unimportant and unnecessary so that I could focus on living the game I'd dreamed up while still living a relatively normal life as a writer, nerd, and gamer.

The best part about all of this? I can teach anybody to do it!

In fact, I've taught thousands of people how to do it, and they're currently on adventures as we speak. We call ourselves The Rebellion—inspired by the Rebel Alliance of Star Wars lore—and I want you to join us. Consider this book a strategy guide for your game of life, and the manual for membership in The Rebellion. Not only will I be sharing the exact blueprint you can follow to start living your life like the video game, book, and movie characters you love, but I'll also share dozens of stories from our ragtag community of Rebels: unexpected heroes, underdogs, and unlikely adventurers who have done the same. I'm going to share with you:

* How a seventh-grade teacher visited five continents in the past 4 years without taking on a single dollar of debt.
* How a single dad took his love of anime and gamified his martial arts practice to connect and train with his son.
* How a Rebel living below the poverty line got his act together, with the goal of competing in his first adventure race on the other side of the country.
* How a divorced 55-year-old retired firefighter took control of her life and built an app company.
* How a Filipino college student used a secret powerup to find the best job on campus and overcame a fear of public performance to join a public dance group.
* How a clinical hematology specialist retooled his life around exploring nature, volunteering at a suicide prevention hotline, and even scoring a major role in a musical.

These Rebels, along with many others, have built their day-to-day lives in varied ways, and I'm so excited to share their stories with you. Throughout this book, you'll find Rebel Spotlights that highlight each person, along with their day job, alter ego, video-game profession, and how they have leveled up their lives. It's been fun to watch people from every possible background level up.

However, if you're reading that list and wondering how the heck you're going to make such drastic changes from the life you're currently not happy with, you're not alone. We've all been there. Going through the motions rather than enjoying each day. Counting down to the weekend, counting down to next year, counting down to some mythical "when things slow down" date in the future (that doesn't actually exist) until we can start to do all of the things we truly want to do. When we're drifting mindlessly through our lives rather than actively participating in them, we often look to escape when real life becomes unfulfilling or too daunting.

It's the equivalent of Bilbo Baggins, the hero in J.R.R. Tolkien's *The Hobbit*, quietly living out an existence in his hobbit-hole, avoiding anything that could be dangerous, adventurous, or exciting. We know something is missing in our lives, or we dream of something more, but aren't quite able to identify what that is. And yet it seems like year after year goes by with nothing actually changing, and pretty soon we're looking back and asking ourselves, "What the heck happened?" If any of this is hitting close to home, that life is passing you by, then this is the book for you.

I'm going to show you exactly how to live a life you can be proud of, how to have adventures that will inspire your friends, and how to finally start doing all the things you said you would do eventually but never seem to find the time for. Whether it's traveling more, losing weight, running a marathon, learning a new instrument, starting a website, or anything in between, The Rebellion would love to have you.

Now, when you join The Rebellion, there's a list of rules we choose to abide by. Our first rule is that we don't care where you come from, only where you're going. Whether you're an 18-year-old high school senior trying to figure out what the heck to do with your life or a 55-year-old divorcée yearning for something more, I'm excited to help.

The next rule? When you join, you join for life. We've got a lot of work to do, but I promise it's going to be a lot of fun. All I ask is that you trust me, and that when I ask you to take a leap of faith, you jump. Our focus is going to be on daily improvement, finding a way to be a bit better, a bit closer to our goal each and every day. But it starts here and now. As Morpheus tells Neo in the movie *The Matrix*:

"This is your last chance. After this, there is no turning back. You take the blue pill—the story ends, you wake up in your bed and believe whatever you want to believe. You take the red pill—you stay in Wonderland and I show you how deep the rabbit hole goes."

Shall we take the red pill?

SECTION 1

THE CALL
TO
ADVENTURE

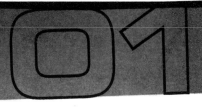

LEAVING THE SHIRE

IN A HOLE IN THE GROUND THERE LIVED A HOBBIT. NOT A NASTY, DIRTY, WET HOLE, FILLED WITH THE ENDS OF WORMS AND AN OOZY SMELL, NOR YET A DRY, BARE, SANDY HOLE WITH NOTHING IN IT TO SIT DOWN ON OR TO EAT: IT WAS A HOBBIT-HOLE, AND THAT MEANS COMFORT. —J.R.R. TOLKIEN, THE HOBBIT

I f you're wondering how I went from risk-averse nerd to globe-trotting Indiana Jones, it started in 2007 with a panic attack.

It happened while I was sitting on a plane flying home to San Diego, but it wasn't because I was afraid of flying. The issue was that I dreamed of traveling to far-off lands, doing exciting things, and living an epic life full of adventure, but my reality was drastically different from the dreams taking place in my head. After spending all day at a job I was ill-suited for, I would spend every night and weekend hiding behind my computer screen, emptying hour after hour into video games in order to escape an existence that could best be described as dull and directionless. I ate the same foods, did the same boring things, and put off any adventure and growth of any kind until things in my life were "less busy." I felt like I was having a midlife crisis at the age of 23. As Ben Franklin said, "Some people die at 25 and aren't buried until 75." I felt like he was speaking to me.

I wanted more out of life, but had no idea how to make it happen. I continued to escape into video games, books, and movies to live life through the eyes of characters whose lives seemed (and were) more exciting than mine. I zoned out every night in front of a screen, got drunk on the weekends to forget the previous week, and dreaded Sunday nights because I knew I'd have to wake up early the next morning and go back to a reality that I despised. I thought back to my youth and tried to figure out where things went wrong.

I had a very normal childhood. Well, if you can call growing up in a town called Sandwich "normal." To answer your first two questions, yes, our police cars say "Sandwich Police" on them, and no, our high school mascot is not a sandwich. As a young child, I had an overly active imagination, and split my free time equally between playing games like *The Legend of Zelda* and exploring my backyard as if I was Link, the tunic-wearing hero of that game. I honestly felt like I grew up alongside Link, watching him jump from a 2D sprite in *A Link to the Past* to a fully realized 3D badass in *The Ocarina of Time*, widely considered the greatest games of all time.

And then came my four years at Sandwich High School; as a sophomore I stood a towering 5'1", on year #3 of braces, and I somehow managed to get the acne that comes with puberty without the accompanying growth spurt. Finally, my exceptionally tall father's genetics kicked in, and I grew to 5'11" by the time I finished my junior year. The braces came off and two rounds of Accutane treatments helped clear up my skin. I even tried out for the varsity basketball team, as my brother was captain and I prided myself on trying really hard. Unfortunately, all the effort in the world couldn't mask the fact that I wasn't very good, and I got cut. Thus, the only two sports I ended up playing in high school were those generally recommended for geriatrics: golf and tennis. It was right around this time, too, that I managed to fall in love and spend all of my free time hopelessly addicted. Her name?

EverQuest.

For the unfamiliar, *EverQuest* is an immensely popular online multiplayer video game like *World of Warcraft* in which a world of wizards, warriors, and dragons reside. If you grew up playing Dungeons & Dragons, think of this like its video game equivalent without a dungeon master. I didn't have my driver's license or a girlfriend, so my weekends and summer nights were spent exploring in a different way. Rather than actively exploring my backyard or new parts of town, I explored the game world of Norrath as Morphos Novastorm, an Erudite Wizard. No longer did I need to use my imagination to fill in the gaps, because Norrath had it all: massively high peaks, deep dark oceans full of secrets, deserted islands, haunted houses, caves, castles, and everything in between.

What had begun as a fun way to blow off some steam after school or work quickly became an addiction. I specifically remember a few nights after marathon gaming sessions in which I would quietly try to sneak up to bed so as to not wake my parents, only to bump into my dad who was getting ready for work. Sorry, Dad. There were quite a few days during the summer in which I stayed up all night trying to complete a particularly challenging quest, only to realize it was already time to go work a 12-hour shift at my summer day job, stocking shelves in busy supermarkets for Coca-Cola. It paid great, but boy was I miserable.

Although I dedicated a lot of my time to gaming after school and on weekends, I made sure to keep a strong focus on my academics, too. Having an older brother who graduated second in his class paved a nice path for me to put all sorts of unnecessary pressure on myself to follow in his footsteps. I joined every club I could, served on student council, got the best grades I could, and managed to graduate second in my small class as well. Eventually, I chose to attend Vanderbilt University in Nashville, Tennessee. I didn't know much about the school other than the fact that it had a great reputation and nicer weather than the Northeast, so when they offered me a decent academic scholarship I decided to visit the campus and instantly fell in love with it.

My four years of college progressed rather quickly. I wasn't sure what I wanted to be when I grew up—and I still don't know—so I bounced between majors before finally settling on economics. I loved college. Not because I could party all the time—I actually didn't start drinking until my senior year. I loved college because I had freedom and a computer with max specifications that could run the best games at the highest resolution. My roommates and I pooled our money together to buy a big TV and every available game system, and we spent hours upon hours playing *Super Smash Bros., Halo, Mario Kart, Resident Evil,* and every role-playing game (RPG) we could find. It was in the fall of my junior year that *EverQuest 2* was released, and my love affair with online video games began anew. In between classes, after class, before going out on weekends (or instead of going out on weekends), and instead of writing papers, my time went into leveling up my character in the newly designed Norrath.

As graduation neared and I still had zero plans for my future, my brother Jack contacted me from a frozen Chicago to tell me he wanted me to move with him to San Diego, California. Because I had no other plans, I quickly consented, and after graduating I moved out West and took the highest paying job I could find in an industry that would have me: construction equipment rental and sales. I figured, "How hard could it be? I like talking to people, and both of my parents are in sales!"

We lived 20 yards from the beach, I surfed when I could, I had a company car, a steady salary, and a job that kept me busy, and I was miserable. Every morning hit me like a sack of hammers, and I quickly counted down the minutes until my shift ended and I could go home. I certainly don't mean to knock the construction industry or sales, it's just that it only took me a few days to realize that I was simply mismatched and terrible at it. Fortunately, I had a wallet full of money and a computer that could run *EverQuest 2.* So afternoons were spent playing video games, weekends were spent getting drunk at bars or drinking and playing *EverQuest,* and Sundays were reserved for walking along the beach, fighting back tears, wondering what's wrong, and asking myself, "Am I really supposed to be this unhappy for the next forty years?"

Even though I wasn't great at my job, I tried to tough things out and did so for over a year, hoping things would improve. Spoiler alert: they didn't. In fact, things got worse! My boss had GPS devices installed on our sales trucks, and I vividly remember one morning getting a phone call from the boss man at 7:05 a.m. "Steve," he said. "I can see that your truck is still parked in front of your house. Why haven't you left yet? Your day should start at seven a.m." Not to be outsmarted, I simply drove from job site to job site, quickly made my sales pitches and usually got rejected, and then sat in my truck and read Harry Potter novels for 20 minutes before repeating the process until my work day was over. As an overachiever in high school, I couldn't help but think about how far I had fallen in just a few short years. Honestly, I'm thankful I was so miserable and mismatched with that job, as a somewhat happier existence might not have spurred me to action!

SUNDAYS WERE RESERVED FOR WALKING ALONG THE BEACH, FIGHTING BACK TEARS, WONDERING WHAT'S WRONG, AND ASKING MYSELF, "AM I REALLY SUPPOSED TO BE THIS UNHAPPY FOR THE NEXT FORTY YEARS?"

Now, it was right around this time that I had the aforementioned panic attack on the airplane and decided some adventure was in order. I had just spent an amazing weekend back in Nashville with all of my college friends for a reunion, and, for the first time in over a year, I was truly happy.

I walked off that plane a different man and decided I needed to make a change. I reached out to the friends I had just visited, who informed me they were in search of a third roommate for their new apartment in Atlanta. I woke up the next morning, marched into my brother's room, and let him know I had to move to Atlanta as quickly as possible. Fortunately he was incredibly supportive and helped me begin my job search; my boss was less enthusiastic about the idea.

While checking Craigslist, I stumbled across a posting online for a job that required "creativity, a love of music, and willingness to travel." Even though it was a subentry level position, it was with a company named Sixthman that gave me a warm fuzzy feeling. Sixthman produces floating music festivals by chartering cruise ships and filling them up with music acts of various genres.

During the interview process, I was asked which movie had inspired me the most. Having just gone through a perfectly mundane and boring existence out in California, I went on and on about the movie *The Shawshank Redemption*, in which an inmate refuses to let his prison walls beat him down or change him. As luck would have it, *Shawshank* also happened to be the favorite movie of the owner of the company, and I was brought on as a marketing assistant.

Although I earned less than half of what I'd been making out in San Diego, I absolutely loved the job: I worked with people I admired, I made an immediate impact, and my day-to-day office life always built up to an amazing event with incredible musicians. On one cruise, the company tasked me to write about my experiences onboard: my first creative writing assignment. After sharing my work with the company, I was soon put in charge of the company blog, and I fell in love with using written words to share stories and inspire people to live a life of fun.

Now, although I enjoyed my time on these cruises and in the office, whenever it was possible I still poured dozens of hours into *EverQuest 2*. Deep down, I knew something was still missing. I no longer dreaded Mondays, and I had plenty of things in my life to look forward to, but something inside me told me my future still lay elsewhere. A year prior I had purchased the domain NerdFitness .com, a half-baked idea I had to help nerds like myself not make all of the mistakes I had made in the gym trying to get healthy. I enjoyed exercising, but increasingly saw my fitness and my dreams of building a company get put on the back burner as more and more time was required of my wizard, Morphos Novastorm.

And then fate intervened again. While on a taxing dungeon raid in *EverQuest*, the fan in the computer I had built burned out, and many of the internal components fried. It was then that I made a commitment to myself: because I lacked the money to fix or replace the computer, I wouldn't allow myself to play *EverQuest* again until I had actually done something with Nerd Fitness. I spent the next 18 months leading a double life; during the day I was the marketing guy for Sixthman, while at night I worked on Nerd Fitness—writing articles, connecting with readers, and helping others make better food and exercise decisions. I didn't get much sleep, but I spent most of my days smiling, happy, and freaking wired: I had finally found my path. True growth and adventure had thus far eluded me, but it was getting closer by the day. And that's when my life started to get interesting.

After those 18 months working on Nerd Fitness on nights and weekends, it became clear to me that my destiny and future lay with the website and community I was building. So I made the brutally difficult decision to walk away from a great job and devote myself full-time to helping people live healthier lives. Fortunately, my boss understood completely and asked how he could support my dream. To this day Andy and I remain great friends, and I count him as a trusted advisor. I picked up odd jobs here and there to make ends meet while Nerd Fitness grew—including pushing around heavy concert gear, working beer stands at festivals, painting soundstage floors late into the night—and put a focus on the true life I wanted to build for myself.

Then, one day it hit me. Instead of continuing to play *Ever-Quest* in my free time or dumping more time into games, books, and movies, I wanted to turn my life into a game. I still lived a double life, but things had changed. By day, I worked on NerdFitness .com, spending hours at my laptop writing articles and connecting with people. By night I could become adventurous Steve Kamb, actively planning crazy experiences that would take me out of my comfortable hobbit-hole and away to far-off lands, into life-changing moments of growth and adventure.

Screw bucket lists—they're boring, unoriginal, and few people ever cross anything off them. My game would be called "The Epic Quest of Awesome." With this game, I drew inspiration from all of my favorite movies, video games, and books. I developed a system that allowed me to gain experience points, accomplish quests, complete missions, and literally level up my life. I created a list of things that would challenge me physically (for example: completing a handstand push-up or learning a martial art), challenge me mentally (learning a new musical instrument or language), push me outside of my comfort zone (eating exotic foods like crocodile or visiting a foreign country where I didn't speak the language), create financial independence (building my own business and paying off my student loans), and even helping others (volunteering my time and donating to charity).

> I'D BECOME SO INSPIRED BY THE GAMES AND MOVIES I LOVED THAT I DECIDED TO GO ON A LIFE-CHANGING, GLOBE-TROTTING QUEST OF MY OWN TO SEE IF THIS WHOLE "LIFE IS A GAME" IDEA COULD TRULY BE ACTUALIZED.

Then, I looked at a map of the world as if it were a video game world. South America became the "Jungle Zone"; Africa became the "Desert Zone." I identified all the missions, goals, and quests I wanted to accomplish in each "zone" that would help me live the life I wanted. I even created a leveling system in which each time I crossed a goal off my list, I would receive experience points toward the next level. Whenever I gained enough experience, I leveled up. Ultimately, I modeled my life and free time off the game mechanics that used to keep me chained to my desk. Instead of leveling up in *EverQuest*, I could level up in real life. And then I did.

I'd become so inspired by the games and movies I loved that I decided to go on a life-changing, globe-trotting quest of my own to see if this whole "Life is a Game" idea could truly be actualized. I sold almost everything I owned, packed the rest into a backpack, and set off on a trip around the globe that would make Marco Polo blush. I hit over a dozen countries, completed a few dozen quests, said, "What the $%#@ am I doing?" at least a hundred times, and returned home a changed nerd.

I now live a life not unlike Indiana Jones. During the day I live a regular existence working on Nerd Fitness, researching and writing articles to inspire and educate people who want to retake control of their lives. I keep myself physically fit, fill up my afternoons with activities that challenge me, and use my nights to start planning my next adventure. I go to bed proud and wake up excited.

As in any video game, I started at Level 1—a complete newbie—and leveled up from there. I identified the first few goals that I could accomplish more easily than others, which gave me the confidence and freedom to tackle more difficult challenges. I hacked my productivity to get more done in less time, freeing myself up to build my business, stay in shape, conduct research, and still have time to play the occasional video game.

While on my journey, I've connected with elite players and mentors who could provide me with guidance, like Cash McLaughlin. Cash, my best friend since first grade, joined me on my first international trip to Peru to help me build confidence to start traveling more. I also collaborated with other heroes and friends and we all enjoyed (and continue to enjoy) helping each other with our respective missions. I even make sure I have a team to push me to be better by keeping me accountable.

I've hacked my fitness to identify the most important exercises and nutrition decisions that would get me in the best shape of my life, despite not having access to a gym and having a chaotic travel schedule. I've constructed a training regimen that allows me to try any activity I want without worrying about my body breaking down or being ill-equipped to handle its physical demands.

Along with hacking myself physically, I've hacked my brain, too. I actively seek out small failures to learn from so that I can succeed at big missions. I seek out challenges that scare the crap out of me, which has led to jumping out of airplanes, leaping off bridges, and giving talks in front of large groups of people despite wanting to vomit seconds beforehand. And everything I've done

CONTINUED ON PAGE 14

REBEL HERO

★ ★ ★ ★ ★ ★

NAME: Ariel Strong   **AGE:** 57

HOMETOWN: Phoenix, AZ

I had nearly given up on getting fit again because of an injury and was depressed that I could no longer work as a firefighter. I stumbled upon The Rebellion and decided that it was worth another try. Since then, I've totally changed my health and life. Using the free six-week challenges on the site, I went from drinking 3 or more cans of soda a day to being soda-free for more than a year now. Group role-playing through the Nerd Fitness challenges and mini-challenges from the Rangers Guild has helped me lose weight and get stronger and more flexible. I'm finally able to hike again!

Those changes have rippled out into the rest of my life. Better eating and exercise led to losing weight which has led to more confidence, which led me to participate in a Startup Weekend, which led to winning an award for my "Fight the Fire" game app prototype. That showed me that I could combine my nerdy love of games and technology with my fire-fighting knowledge to create a whole new career for myself. I now have a fledgling game development startup at a local co-working space where I am surrounded by nerds and gamers and people who know the value of imagination and creative play.

Nerd Fitness has given me tools to use to improve other areas of my life, as well. Role playing my character, "Shadow

SPOTLIGHT

DAY JOB: *App Developer*

ALTER EGO: *Shadow Lion*   **CLASS:** *Ranger*

Lion," has fueled my creativity in writing and led to friendships with other creative nerds. The community in The Rebellion forums is wonderful and is a crucial part of success in leveling up one's life. It is an added bonus that it spans the globe and I have nerd friends from around the world. We support each other and cheer each other on; we help each other get through the tough times. I never realized that digital connections could be that strong.

I still have a long way to go, but The Rebellion has given me hope that someday I will get back out on a wildland fire engine again, even if only as a volunteer. And in the meantime, I have an epic quest, fun work with a worthy mission, and friends for the journey! What more could a nerd want?

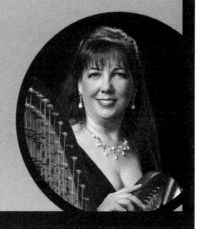

that has improved my life over the past five years, I've learned and adapted from the very movie and video game characters that used to keep me "prisoner" at my desk and on my couch.

I realize that turning one's life into a video game might sound silly to some. But video games, for the tens of millions of us who have grown up playing them, are a fundamental part of our lives and how we see the world. The creators of the games we love know exactly how to hook us with a compelling story, deliver engaging game mechanics to make us happy, and give us frequent challenges and rewards that keep us coming back for more.

And that is what I will teach you: exactly how to take the things you love and use them as inspiration and education to help you level up your own life. The Rebellion is glad to have you, and I can't wait to see what game you create for yourself. It starts with taking imperfect action.

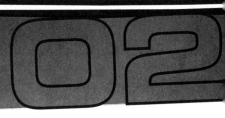

THE CAUTIONARY TALE OF THE UNDERPANTS GNOMES

GOTTA GO TO WORK, WORK, WORK, WORK! WE WON'T STOP 'TIL WE HAVE UNDERPANTS!

—THE UNDERPANTS GNOMES, SOUTH PARK

Before we leave the comfy confines of our hobbit-hole in the Shire for a life of adventure, I must first tell you a cautionary tale. I'm sure right now you're all fired up and ready to turn your life into a video game. But I must warn you: if you're not careful, you could look back years from now and realize that all you've really done is collect a giant pile of underpants.

I promise this will make sense.

It all starts with the show *South Park*. In the small town of South Park, Colorado, a group of small underpants gnomes sneak into people's houses during the middle of the night and steal their underpants, delivering them to a massive underground chamber each night. They even have a theme song that they sing while working: imagine the seven dwarves of Snow White fame, but with more underpants: "Gotta go to work, work, work, work! We won't stop 'til we have underpants!"

You might wonder why these gnomes are stealing people's underpants, which is a valid question. It turns out they're collecting underpants because it's part of their master plan to build a highly successful business. However, when a gnome is questioned as to why he is collecting underpants, he always says, "Collecting underpants is just Phase 1!"

When somebody inevitably asks, "What's Phase 2?" every gnome replies with "Phase 3 is profit!" So they know collecting underpants is Phase 1 and that Phase 3 is profit, but Phase 2 is a complete mystery. Nobody has any idea what it is! They consult their business plan, and Phase 2 is just a giant question mark. So, rather than trying to figure it out, these gnomes spend all day and all night dutifully collecting underpants without having any clue

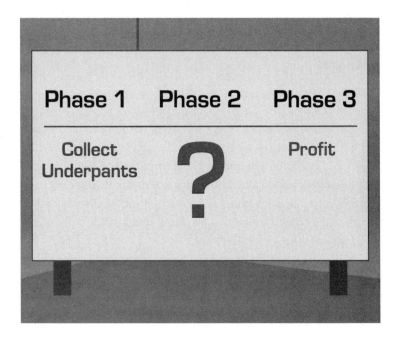

as to how to move onto Phase 2, which would then eventually get them to the all-important Phase 3.

Whether you realize it or not, you are an underpants gnome! Any time you read an inspiring news story, watch a YouTube video of somebody doing something amazing, or read a book like this one that encourages you to make changes in your life, you are collecting underpants. In fact, most of us spend all day reading, watching, or listening to things and then going, "Whoa, it would be so cool if I could do that!" Then we dutifully move on to the next nugget of knowledge or inspiration that makes us say, "I'd love to do that some day!" Each time we do this, we are contributing to our pile of underpants. Whether it's scanning a fitness site for advice on completing a marathon, reading a phrase book to better learn French, watching a video of somebody doing parkour, attending a TEDx conference and learning about volunteering opportunities in Africa, or even just reading this very book, we are all making mental notes of the things we'd like to do. This is the equivalent of collecting a pile of underpants.

Welcome to Phase 1.

Phase 3 is what you hope to accomplish after starting to build your pile: your life when you are firing on all cylinders. You are embarking on adventures, you are challenging yourself, you wake up excited, you feel purpose each and every day. Which brings me to the point of this chapter: when you join The Rebellion, you learn to dominate Phase 2. You can spend all day every day learning and collecting and researching. You could read this book so many times that you memorize it cover to cover. In fact, you could become the best information gatherer in the entire world, for hundreds of subjects. Gathering information is a great start—Phase 1 is a crucial part of the equation. After all, it's tough to solve a problem if you don't study it, and it's tough to work out a solution without understanding what you hope to accomplish with it. However, if you only focus on Phase 1, all you'll be left with is a big pile of underpants!

Phase 2 is about figuring out what to do with that knowledge you've been collecting so that you can advance to Phase 3, which

> THIS BOOK IS PHASE 1, AND IF YOU'RE NOT CAREFUL IT'S EASY TO READ AND PUT OFF TAKING ACTION UNTIL YOUR LIFE GETS "LESS BUSY." THE TRUTH IS THAT THERE IS NEVER A BETTER TIME TO START THAN RIGHT NOW. I CAN PROMISE YOU THAT "EVENTUALLY" NEVER HAPPENS, AND THAT "SOMEDAY" NEVER COMES.

could be health, love, happiness, adventure, or any combination of the things that remind us it's a damn good day to be alive. People who dominate Phase 2 are action-takers. They understand that collecting a few underpants and then immediately trying to do things with that knowledge is a much faster path to Phase 3 than just collecting more and more underpants!

Phase 2 is about learning, trying, failing, backtracking, trying again, and learning even more. Phase 2 is about going for your first hike despite not having the best gear. Phase 2 is about attempting your first push-up even if it's ugly. Phase 2 is about trying to build your first mobile app instead of reading yet another book about programming. Phase 2 is about conversing on Skype with a native speaker of the language you are trying to learn (in broken phrases, if necessary) instead of reading yet another book on that language. Phase 2 is about approaching somebody you'd like to meet rather than reading yet another book on social skills. This book is Phase 1, and if you're not careful it's easy to read and put off taking action until your life gets "less busy."

The truth is that there is never a better time to start than right now. I can promise you that "eventually" never happens, and that "someday" never comes. I receive emails every day from people who say things like: "I've done the research, I know what I'm supposed to do, but I don't have the motivation to start on my journey. Can you give me some please?"

Unfortunately, I can't. We'll cover the fallacy of motivation later in the book, but for now I'll tell you that the desire to change, live better, look better, feel better, and then have the guts to try things out and see what works (essentially, what you do with your pile of underpants) has to come from within you. Phase 2 is about the ability to fail repeatedly and continue to attempt new and different ways to succeed. As Winston Churchill declared, "Success is the ability to go from one failure to another with no loss of enthusiasm." And don't worry, if the idea of failure or the unknown scares you, we're going to solve that problem, too.

People often ask me how I built a life around my love of games and helping people get fit. It's simple: I started. I was working a normal job, I lived a normal life, and then I read a few books (which I'll share with you later) to give myself the shot of confidence I needed to start making some changes. Then I started writing and helping people in my spare time. I didn't spend more money on blogging classes, Internet marketing books, SEO strategy, or writing courses (that's a lot of expensive underpants). Instead, I started writing crappy articles that got less and less crappy with each publication. I put my focus on helping people and learning how to make more of an impact with my writing, made plenty of mistakes, and learned from them. Years later, here I am.

Ask Jim Bathurst of BeastSkills.com how he became the amazing gymnastics guru he is today: he taught himself! He read some books and watched videos, he observed other people doing the things he wanted to do, and then he went out and tried to do them! He fell, busted up his body repeatedly, and struggled at the beginning, but over time and bit by bit he improved—and now he does one-handed handstands and teaches people this stuff for a living.

I'm going to let you in on a secret: spend 10 percent of your time and effort on Phase 1, and 90 percent on trying out the new things you are learning. Paint your first terrible picture. Write the first chapter of a book that will never be read. Ask somebody out and get shot down. Save money for a trip and book the damn thing. Start a crappy blog. Record a few awful podcasts. Pluck a few wrong notes on a guitar. Pronounce words incorrectly in a foreign language.

Why?

Because you're actually doing something! Nothing comes of collecting more underpants other than a bigger pile of underpants.

Until you learn what to do with them, you'll only ever have a pile of underpants and never arrive at the happiness you are seeking. This book will guide you from Phase 1 to Phase 3, but I cannot complete Phase 2 for you: You're gonna have to get up off your ass and do that yourself.

"But, Steve," you might be thinking, "I don't know where to start." As in any game, there will be times when you see many paths ahead of you, and you have no clue which one you need to take. I hear you, and I know that it can be overwhelming. However, the worst thing you can do is sit down on the ground and complain that you don't know what to do. More information at this point isn't going to help, either. That's just more underpants! Instead, why not just make an educated guess, pick a path, and see how things work out? Think of it like becoming the main character in a Choose Your Own Adventure book—it's tough to find out what happens if you don't turn the page.

Speaking of books, my favorite example of this comes from J.R.R. Tolkien's *The Fellowship of the Ring*. The gang is lost in a cave and stumbles across a path that leads in three different directions. After sitting in that spot for hours, unsure of which path to take, how do they eventually decide? Gandalf simply decides that the air doesn't smell so foul down one of the paths.

When you are faced with a similar decision, just start. It's going to be tough for us to save Middle Earth if we never leave the hobbit-hole, right? It's going to be tough to hack the Matrix if we take the blue pill and do nothing. You can't save the world, and you can't find the end of the maze by sitting on your butt wondering which path to take. Research and a logical decision-making process helps, but sometimes you just have to move.

So other than reading this book, do yourself a favor and don't collect any more underpants for the time being. As you are reading, don't be afraid to put it down and get started and come back to it as you find different paths along your journey. As Ellie says in Pixar's *Up*, "Adventure is out there!" Let's go find it.

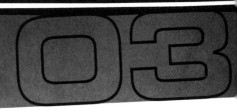

READY PLAYER ONE

IT'S A DANGEROUS BUSINESS, FRODO, GOING OUT YOUR DOOR. YOU STEP ONTO THE ROAD, AND IF YOU DON'T KEEP YOUR FEET, THERE'S NO KNOWING WHERE YOU MIGHT BE SWEPT OFF TO.

—BILBO BAGGINS, THE LORD OF THE RINGS

If you choose to believe it, today is a crucial turning point in your life. Think back to your favorite story, myth, or tale. They all start somewhere ordinary, with a normal person or child of humble beginnings, who goes on to do something great:

Star Wars: A long time ago, in a galaxy far, far away . . .

The Hunger Games: May the odds be ever in your favor.

The Hobbit: In a hole in the ground there lived a hobbit.

Harry Potter: The boy who lived.

We all love origin stories, because we get to see our heroes as normal people: Bruce Wayne before he became Batman, Natasha Romanova before she became Black Widow, Steve Rogers before he became Captain America. It turns out you're currently at the beginning of your origin story, too. We all have to start somewhere, and we'll need to go through our own journey full of ups and downs before we can return a changed man or woman. None of that can happen, however, if we don't heed the call for adventure.

I'll never forget the first time I saw the original *Star Wars Episode IV: A New Hope.* To this day, watching Luke Skywalker walk out of his home on Tatooine with the binary sunset in the distance, as John Williams's epic score plays, sends chills down my spine. I imagined I was Luke, and it was destined that I would bring peace and balance to the Galaxy. He grew up on a farm, I grew up in suburbia; he went on to do great things, so why couldn't I?

When we're stuck in a crappy desk job (or even worse, a perfectly comfortable but unfulfilling job!) or in a relationship that makes us miserable, we daydream about getting pulled into another dimension where we can live the lives we were meant to live, and exciting things happen to us. Most importantly, along with an escape, these stories give us hope when things aren't going so well:

* Luke Skywalker worked on a farm and then went on to save the Galaxy!
* The Goonies were a group of kids in a podunk town and they found a pirate ship full of treasure practically in their backyard.
* Katniss was a regular girl who went on to lead a revolution against the oppressive rulers of Panem!

We all know how important hope is. The movie *The Shawshank Redemption* said it best: "Hope is a good thing. Maybe the best of things, and no good thing ever dies." Belief in these epic journeys gives us the hope we need to struggle and persevere through a dull existence to reach the good stuff. More than ever, we need these stories to endure the low points in our lives.

Now, believing in these stories as children is encouraged by our parents; we're told it's good to have an active imagination, and that we can be whatever we want to be when we grow up. We're encouraged to read, to make believe, to tell the world we're going to be an astronaut or a cowboy or a magician. As we get older, however, it becomes easier and easier to accept mediocrity. We're told to accept our place in the world, our expanding waistline, our boring job. We're told to accept a life that leaves us unfulfilled because that's just the way things are. If things don't work out, it's because life isn't fair. Sure, we had hopes and dreams back in the day, but this is reality. There's no time to travel, no time to write that novel, no time to learn the guitar, no time to find happiness. If we're overweight, unhappy, in a dead-end job, in a relationship that sucks, or we're going nowhere with our lives, that's just tough luck. We're told to suck it up and deal with it. To be realistic. That's just the way it is.

> WE CAN HOPE FOR A BETTER EXISTENCE—WE CAN WANT HAPPINESS AND ADVENTURE IN OUR LIVES—BUT IN ORDER FOR THAT TO HAPPEN, WE NEED TO HEED THE CALL WHEN IT COMES KNOCKING. HOPE WITHOUT ACTION RESULTS IN NO CHANGE.

Only it isn't. We can hope for a better existence—we can want happiness and adventure in our lives—but in order for that to happen, we need to heed the call when it comes knocking. Hope without action results in no change.

Star Wars would have been mighty boring if it was a trilogy about Luke as a farmer—no offense intended to interplanetary farmers. Harry Potter would have sucked if it was seven books of him getting pummeled by his cousin Dudley. *The Goonies* would have been a crappy movie if they had found that treasure map and then went back to watching Chunk do the Truffle Shuffle.

Hope needs to be combined with action for the story to progress. A call needs to be answered. Adventure can start anytime, anywhere, but it has to start. You're in that part of your story now.

Life is meant to be lived on your own terms.

That's a simple statement, yet it's one we often lose sight of. We do what we think we're supposed to, what "the right move" for us is at this point in our lives, or what makes the most sense on paper, instead of doing what will allow us to grow and find true happiness. We often decide to follow a particular path to make our parents happy or to appease our spouses, because we think we have no better alternative. Or worse, we do it simply because everybody else is doing it. Heck, we often pick a path because it's the one that's easiest or causes the least amount of discomfort! But if we're not careful, too many of these seemingly insignificant decisions can lead to a life that's merely endured, not enjoyed.

> WE OFTEN PICK A PATH BECAUSE IT'S THE ONE THAT'S EASIEST OR CAUSES THE LEAST AMOUNT OF DISCOMFORT! BUT IF WE'RE NOT CAREFUL, TOO MANY OF THESE SEEMINGLY INSIGNIFICANT DECISIONS CAN LEAD TO A LIFE THAT'S MERELY ENDURED, NOT ENJOYED.

In the book, *The Top Five Regrets of the Dying*, the #1 regret voiced by those on their deathbeds, having the crystal-clear ability to look back at what they had done or not done over the course of their lives, is that they wished they'd had the courage to live lives true to themselves, as opposed to the lives others expected of them.

Let that sink in for a moment.

These are not philosophical or hypothetical ponderings, but rather real-life reflections from people who know they're down to their last quarter in the arcade, so to speak. These people didn't live the lives they wanted to live; they felt a call to adventure or a call for a path that challenged and fulfilled them, and yet refused the call because they didn't want to ruffle any feathers or were scared of what that path might reveal. They instead chose the easy, safe, nonconflicting path; a life that others expected them to live, and they would give anything now for an extra life or to try again and take the more adventurous route.

Until we develop time machines, older folks will never have

the luxury of trying again, but you can certainly learn from the wisdom of their words. If you want to live a life of adventure, you need to stop thinking of what others want for you, and instead start asking what you want for yourself.

Yes, choosing to live a life you want might cause some issues or confusion among those around you. If both your parents are doctors, there could be tremendous pressure for you to attend med school; if your siblings are all mechanics, then you might be expected to join the family business. Both my parents were in sales, and although they never once pushed me in that direction, I pushed myself in that direction because I knew it would make them happy, and I didn't have a strong desire to focus on anything else. But it turns out we do have a chance to be whatever we want to be, to experience the adventures we've always dreamed of experiencing, but we have to be willing to reach for them and bold enough to hold ourselves to that higher expectation.

That's what I did. It wasn't because I was born adventurous. I simply decided to heed the call when it came knocking—my computer exploding—and I became my own hero. Along my journey, I turned the things that used to hold me back into a blueprint for living a life more amazing than any video game or movie. I then recruited others interested in the same stuff and built a Rebellion of hundreds of thousands of people along the way. I've developed a system and philosophy that altered my life's path through tiny incremental steps and realigned my priorities. It took years of work, plenty of struggle, and more than a few tough moments, but that's all part of the process.

Luke didn't become a Jedi overnight; in fact, Master Yoda initially dismissed him for being too old to begin the training! Katniss didn't possess the innate ability to lead a revolution. Neo had to learn how to become The One. Your journey won't be instant either, and it most likely won't be easy! However, I can promise you it will be rewarding.

You have the potential for greatness inside you, but it needs to be awakened. Luke already had the Force, but needed to train

CONTINUED ON PAGE 28

REBEL HERO

★ ★ ★ ★ ★ ★

NAME: Mandy Fritsch   **AGE:** 25

HOMETOWN: Cincinnati, OH

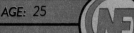

There is both a satisfying calm and grating edge to the predisposition toward introversion. I have experienced extremes of each throughout my short life, fluctuating between determinism and self-doubt. What I am describing is living with mental illness (such a weird phrase). With it, it's hard to envision a future without some sort of debilitation.

What I have learned, with great influence from The Rebellion, is to put on the hard hat and use my strengths to level up my life. I stumbled upon the blog as a senior undergrad. I mulled over the dietary and exercise suggestions that opposed what I witnessed while working as a tech/crew manager at my school's rec (it involved hours on the elliptical and starving). Never really a fan of this, I committed, after hours of Internet research, to trying out a healthier diet and focusing on strength training.

Following the Nerd Fitness philosophy, I made impressive gains that fall. Almost as enjoyable was the process of tracking the workouts and changes. Many can attest to the spreadsheets that litter my walls. I was in amateur-statistician heaven. Then the breaking point. I had been (pretty effectively) fighting another mental episode, with a lot of reassurance from Steve's posts in my journey. But in January, my best friend was killed in a car accident, and the devastation was extreme. This trigger, combined with some gaps in my treatment, landed me in the inpatient psych ward. I was at ground zero. But The Rebellion helped me back up.

SPOTLIGHT

DAY JOB: *R&D Microbiologist*

ALTER EGO: *Oracle* **CLASS:** *Scout*

Released, I was back on campus. I found a job, 7 miles away. Carless, this meant I could either wait for the bus every day, or try to ride my bike. Inspired by the stories of other Rebels, I got on the saddle of my Schwinn cruiser and pedaled the whole way to the pool. Exhausted, I walked into a 10-hour shift. And then biked back. After a couple weeks, I began to enjoy racing my times on the trail. I started expanding my riding territory to accomplish a once-shelved goal to see all of Columbus's metro parks. Using my calculating nature, I planned routes to each one, as well as estimating times and refueling needs.

I have used a lot of tips from Steve's philosophy on goal setting and social anxiety to continue leveling up. I said "yes" to a date, and have now been with my partner for almost a year. I broke down my large goal of seeing all the national parks into smaller goals, and got to climb to Blue Glacier in Olympic (park #6) this summer. The same methodology went into finishing my first triathlon.

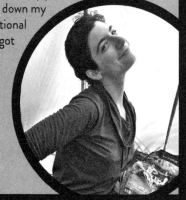

before he could harness that power. Harry was born a wizard but was unaware of his powers until he arrived at Hogwarts. Neo was The One, but until he took that red pill he was a simple programmer, "Thomas Anderson." You are just like these heroes-in-training.

By the time you finish this book, you'll have all the tools, education, inspiration, and support you'll need to take deliberate action toward living a leveled-up life. Not only that, but you'll be using the very characters from your favorite childhood stories and movies to get started. They will teach you how to dream, how to reach, and how to deal with those who don't want you to live out those dreams. All it requires is that you commit to trying new things and making changes that align with what you're hoping to accomplish.

When people ask how things are going, I want you to stop saying "fine, thanks" because that indicates you're just drifting. By the time you've completed your hero's journey, you'll answer that question with, "I'm f@%#ing amazing."

So let's get started. You are the Hero in this story, which means I get to be your mentor. Woohoo! I am Obi-Wan. Gandalf. Morpheus. Professor Dumbledore. I'm going to hold your hand throughout your journey and help you build your Game of Life. If we're going to become what we have the ability to become, we need to get started now. I need you to accept the fact that you're destined for a more important existence than the one you're currently leading. Life is infinitely more fun and rewarding when we level up instead of just existing. There's a superhero version of you waiting to come out, but he or she needs to be rescued. This book is your call to action.

Will you heed the call?

SECTION 2

THE HERO'S JOURNEY

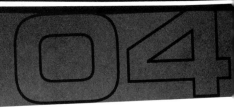

RESCUE YOUR ALTER EGO FROM DOUBTS AND DISBELIEFS

WITH NO POWER COMES NO RESPONSIBILITY. EXCEPT THAT WASN'T TRUE.   *—DAVE LIZEWSKI, KICK-ASS!*

What if I told you that most of your favorite characters—the comic book, movie, book, and video game heroes with whom you most identify and whose adventures you find most exhilarating—all follow a particular story arc that has existed since the dawn of mankind? In *The Hero with a Thousand Faces,* famed mythologist Joseph Campbell introduces the ideas of the Hero's Journey and the Monomyth. In this work, Campbell studies tales dating as far back as Ancient Greece, ancient African tribes, Native American mythology, and medieval ages. What Campbell discovers is that these stories all share the same fundamental structure: A hero ventures forth from the common world into a region of supernatural wonder where fabulous forces are there encountered, and a decisive victory won. The hero comes back from this mysterious adventure with the power to bestow boons on his fellow man.

This idea was later improved by Christopher Vogler in his book, *The Writer's Journey: Mythic Structure for Writers*, in which he describes the Hero's Journey as such:

1. Heroes are introduced to THE ORDINARY WORLD, where
2. They receive the CALL TO ADVENTURE;
3. They are reluctant at first, or REFUSE THE CALL;
4. Are encouraged by a MENTOR to
5. CROSS THE FIRST THRESHOLD and enter the Special World, where
6. They encounter TESTS, ALLIES, and ENEMIES;
7. They APPROACH THE INMOST CAVE, crossing a second threshold,
8. Where they endure the ORDEAL;
9. They take possession of their REWARD and
10. Are pursued on the ROAD BACK to the Ordinary World;
11. They cross the third threshold, experience a RESURREC-TION, and are transformed by the experience.
12. They RETURN WITH THE ELIXIR, a boon, or treasure to benefit the Ordinary World.

As you can see above, the main character is somebody of normal existence who goes through a journey that fundamentally changes him or her as a character. This character learns from a mentor, skeptically accepts the call to leave a comfortable existence, faces trials and tribulations, makes allies and enemies, outsmarts or wins over the guardians of the threshold, struggles to survive/succeed, transforms, and ultimately returns home with an altered/improved outlook on life.

THE HERO'S JOURNEY

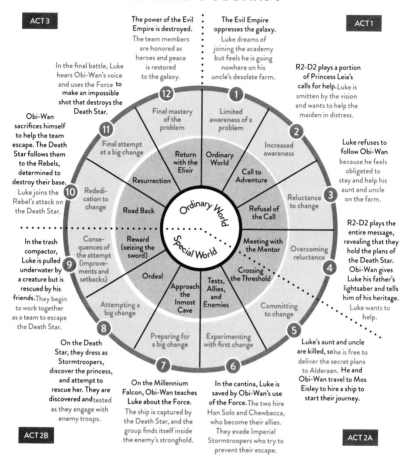

Gray text = inner journey
Red text = outer journey (character transformation)

Now, think of the stories and heroes you love; they all follow this arc. Harry Potter, *Mulan*, Pixar's *Brave*, *Guardians of the Galaxy*, *Cinderella*, *The Hobbit*, *Indiana Jones*, *The Secret Life of Walter Mitty*, *The Lion King*, Star Wars, Iron Man, Thor, Wonder Woman, *The Sword in the Stone*, practically every adventure game, and even Super Mario!

Although the steps occasionally occur out of order, once you understand how the Hero's Journey works you can go back through most any book you've read or movie you've seen and observe it in action. And if you haven't figured it out yet, you're on this journey now. Yes, right now. You are the Hero, and it's time to start building your story arc. You've made it this far, which means you've already accepted that life in the ordinary world isn't fulfilling. You've even met your mentor (yours truly). Once the Call to Adventure comes along (this book), it's time to cross over the threshold to the unknown adventurous life you hope to live. Throughout this book, I'm going to continually refer back to our list of 12 steps in our Hero's Journey as defined by Vogler, reminding you that life is a game or a movie script, you are the hero, and awesome things can happen to you anywhere and everywhere.

In order for us to build the story arc of the life we want to live ourselves, let's begin by examining the existences of superheroes whose story arcs are similar. Just as the Hero's Journey is cyclical, so too are the journeys of superheroes: Tony Stark doesn't live in his Iron Man suit; Bruce Wayne spends as much time being himself as he does as Batman; Indiana Jones doesn't travel the world 24/7, he also teaches archaeology in between bouts of wielding the whip and wearing the fedora. We are going on journeys to follow an arc that takes us in and out of the unknown/adventurous world. I had to go on a Hero's Journey to find my path, and now I get to be your mentor and help you embark on your own.

In other words, I'm giving you permission to live a dual life like any other comic book hero. Yes, you get to have your own origin story, superhero name, and everything, but we need to determine that alter ego first.

CREATING YOUR ORIGIN STORY AND DETERMINING YOUR ALTER EGO

Whether it's Steve Rogers becoming Captain America, Katniss Everdeen becoming the Mockingjay, or Bruce Wayne becoming Batman, it's fun to watch our favorite characters discover their true callings and embrace the supernatural/unknown part of their existences as superheroes. Just as the ordinary caterpillar becomes an extraordinary butterfly, these characters transform spectacularly. And you can, too.

You are at the beginning of your origin story right now, and it's time to build the alter-ego version of yourself that will go through the Hero's Journey and accomplish all the great things you hope to accomplish. The idea of living a life of such adventure may feel intimidating, unlikely, or downright impossible to you at this point, and that's okay! It's okay to be afraid. When I see somebody who's unhealthy, unhappy, or just going through the motions, I see untapped potential, I see someone who is currently "refusing the call." These are people who have the opportunity to embark on the Hero's Journey if they'd just summon the courage to get started.

"But, Steve," you might be thinking, "I'm no hero. And I'm certainly not going to change the world. I just want to feel better about myself and not hate Mondays so much." That's fine. First of all, the best heroes always say, "I'm no hero," so you're in good company there. Next, heroes come in all shapes and sizes, my friend, and superheroes have different types of super powers. Can you be a superhero to your son or daughter? Can you be a superhero to your friends or people who need help? Can you be a superhero to yourself? Remember, you don't need to drastically shake things up—you just need to reprioritize adventure in your alter-ego existence.

Let me share one of my favorite success stories with you:

Thomas Sorensen, an active member of The Rebellion, works as a construction manager in Carson City, Nevada, and he enjoys his regular life. He also happens to be a single parent, and used his love of the Japanese manga *Lone Wolf and Cub* to connect with his son. By combining his love of video games with this particular series, Tom rekindled his love of martial arts to train and create a series of quests for him and his son to complete together. You can read Tom's full story later in this book.

Just as every saga has a beginning, you, too, have an origin story. I want you to take a few minutes now to write out where you are currently and where you plan on going. In other words, what does your real life look like, and how would you spend your time as superhero? If you're not quite sure yet what your super power is or how you'll be spending your free time as a superhero, don't worry. That's what I'm here for. The important thing is to advance your journey by starting. Remember, the more dire your situation is now, the more epic your trip to becoming a Hero will be. The world needs you to become who you were meant to be.

For use as a jumping-off point, here's my own origin story and alter ego:

BY DAY, STEVE KAMB IS AN ORDINARY MAN WITH AN ORDINARY JOB; HE DUTIFULLY WORKS HARD, STRUGGLING WITH EVERYDAY CHALLENGES JUST LIKE ANYBODY ELSE, AND HE SPENDS MOST OF HIS DAYS AT A DESK TRYING TO GROW A BUSINESS. HIS FLAWS ARE THAT HE IS RISK-AVERSE, SHY, A PICKY EATER, AND AFRAID OF QUITE A FEW THINGS—LIKE BUGS AND SNAKES—BUT MORE IMPORTANT, AFRAID OF A LIFE OF BOREDOM. UNKNOWN TO THOSE AROUND HIM, STEVE IS DESTINED FOR BIGGER AND BETTER THINGS, AND NOW HE HAS A SECRET.

STEVE HAS AN ALTER EGO, A SUPERHERO VERSION OF HIMSELF WHO IS CAPABLE OF FAR GREATER THINGS THAN ANYBODY EVER EXPECTED OF HIM. HIS NAME? REBEL ONE. ON NIGHTS AND WEEKENDS, WHEN HE WASN'T AT HIS DAY JOB, STEVE SLOWLY DEVELOPED A CHARACTER WHO COULD DO ALL THE THINGS THE NORMAL STEVE COULDN'T: TRAVEL TO FAR-OFF LANDS, EXPLORE EXOTIC AND DAN-GEROUS LOCATIONS, LEARN NEW SKILLS IN RAPID FASH-ION, AND BE ABLE TO GET INTO OR OUT OF ANY SITUATION. STEVE AND HIS ALTER EGO ARE LIKE A MODERN DAY INDIANA JONES: MAKING DISCOVERIES, HELPING THOSE IN NEED, AND CREATING A LIFETIME OF STORIES AND ADVENTURES. HE DUTIFULLY SPLITS TIME BETWEEN THE TWO LIVES, CYCLING AND TRANSFORMING WITH EACH COMPLETED QUEST OR MISSION.

That's just one example. Ready to create your own? Visit LevelUpYourLife.com to create your own character, write out your origin story, and get ideas from other Rebels.

If you're not sure how to write out your origin story and alter ego, then try this activity: write as if you were looking back on your life at age 99. What did you accomplish in your adventures? What are you known for? Who did you impact? Dream as big and as grand or as small and specific as you'd like to. It's your story, and you get to write the script! I want to know where you are, and where you plan on going.

If you're still struggling with this, I'll hold your hand even more—after all, that's what mentors are for. Here's a *Mad Lib* you can fill in to help get you started:

> [YOUR NAME] LIVED A HUMBLE EXISTENCE AS A
> NERDY [YOUR DAY JOB/OCCUPATION]. LIKE OTHER
> SUPERHERO ORIGIN STORIES, THE HERO STRUGGLED WITH
> [CHARACTER FLAW OR THING MISSING IN YOUR LIFE].
> HOWEVER, AS THE PROPHECIES OF OLD FORETOLD,
> CHANGE WAS COMING. THANKS TO [CALL TO ACTION], AND
> THE AMAZING TUTELAGE OF THE RIDICULOUSLY GOOD-
> LOOKING, CLEVER, AND MODEST MENTOR, STEVE, OUR
> HERO TRANSFORMED, CREATING [ALTER EGO NAME] TO
> PROTECT THE LIVES OF HIS/HER LOVED ONES. ALTHOUGH
> OUR HERO LIVES OUT AN ORDINARY LIFE BY DAY, AT NIGHT
> HE/SHE IS AN ABSOLUTE BADASS, KNOWN FOR [EPIC
> SKILL], [FUN ADVENTUROUS STORY], AND ONE TIME EVEN
> [SOMETHING YOU NEVER THOUGHT YOU'D BE CAPABLE OF].

Just like any superhero, we all have day jobs and obligations. I'm not going to tell you to shirk your duties and move in to a cave to have the adventures laid out in this book (though if that's the path you choose for your story arc, I certainly won't stop you). You don't need to have a bunch of money saved up to start designing an Iron Man suit either. Heroic stories come in all shapes and

CONTINUED ON PAGE 40

REBEL HERO

★ ★ ★ ★ ★ ★

NAME: Ryan Graczkowski　　　**AGE:** 29

HOMETOWN: Raleigh, NC

I love JRPGs (Japanese Role-Playing Games). I really, really do. There's something about the long, slow grind, about the process of building your character from backwoods to badass (although the two are not mutually exclusive!). Before The Rebellion, I was the kind of person who played video games and read lots of stories. Even though I didn't know it, I was soaking up the Hero's Journey, and as corny as it is I grew up thinking that might be me some day. I was a smart kid and I tended to see things a bit differently from everyone else, and I thought if I just had my chance, I'd do something incredible.

When I found The Rebellion in 2011, life wasn't very fun. In a lot of ways, I think I'd given up. My waist was getting bigger, my weight was getting higher, my hair was thinning, and all I could think about was my next opportunity to go grab some fast food. Joining The Rebellion taught me that my life was a game and that I could play it any way I wanted to. So I signed up and started to play.

Last year, I was challenged to get myself up to Boston to participate in a Nerd Fitness meetup and obstacle race with my fellow Rebels. I set aside time to train and budgeted out for the trip accordingly.

Why was this epic? Because I'm poor. As in, I live below the poverty line. When the year started, I was out of a job,

SPOTLIGHT

DAY JOB: Restaurant Associate Trainer

ALTER EGO: Kishi   **CLASS:** Monk

living on unemployment with no real clue what was going to happen. Having this particular quest forced me to really step up, get a job again, and start putting away money to make things happen. And what have I done since then? Well . . .

- I reversed my weight gain. Painfully, with running first, then painlessly when I understood that diet is 80–90% of the battle.

- I discovered that I love running obstacle course races, and have since gone on to run the Warrior Dash, the Rugged Maniac, and a Spartan Sprint. It was after one of these events that I got to meet Steve who made a suprise appearance to show support for us Rebels racing!

- I learned that I love calisthenics, and even though I'm not terribly good at them there's so much to learn!

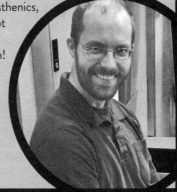

Basically, I learned to get busy living, because I'd already been busy with dying.

sizes, and we need to cycle both through life in the ordinary world and life as a superhero in order to transform.

We're going to have plenty of opportunities to go on quests big and small, near and far, quests that allow us to return transformed to our regular lives and plan out the next quest. But it starts here, with the creation of our origin story and alter ego.

Don't panic if you're not sure this superhero version of yourself is what you really want long term, or that it might change. In many stories, the hero's journey can change paths. Our hero might start out on a treasure hunt, then encounter a love interest who gets kidnapped by an evil villain—the story changes, and so will our lives. Two years into your journey you might have kids, or get married, or change jobs, or get bitten by a radioactive spider, and thus the story can change, too. What's important is that we get started by giving ourselves a direction in which to focus our energy and attention.

Once you've determined what that alter-ego superhero life looks like, every action you take has the opportunity to move you one step closer to your future life as a hero—or further away. Because of this, you need to keep that thought at the front of your mind constantly, and remind yourself daily why you're doing what you're doing. When this happens, you stop worrying about the things you don't have and the things you can't do, and instead focus on the things you can do or the things you will soon be able to do. With each day, with each change, with each small victory, you'll be reinforcing your inevitable future as a badass hero.

The world needs you. Your life as a superhero is about to begin. We've determined the story and arc we want to build, and now we need to build the rest of the story that we're going to live. Oh, and then we need to put a serious plan in place that will allow us to level up our hero and actually complete the missions and quests we're interested in. We're going to go through the whole process step by step, and you're going to make progress every day toward becoming your alter ego. I promise. Nerd's honor.

Let's start now.

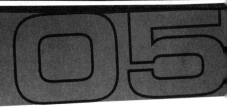

RESIST TEMPTATIONS AND CONVENIENT EXCUSES

HE THAT IS GOOD FOR MAKING EXCUSES IS SELDOM GOOD FOR ANYTHING ELSE. —BENJAMIN FRANKLIN

I f you're a rational human being, then you probably have a tiny voice in your head that tells you why certain things are possible and other things aren't. Most of the time, this is a good voice that can keep you safe. "No, you can't fly if you jump off this ledge," the voice will say; or, "No, you can't eat dog food, that's for the dog, even if it looks tasty." However, this voice can often go too far and actually keep us locked up in a safe, boring existence within our hobbit-holes! This is the voice we need to keep quiet if we're going to turn life into an adventure, because it can derail us if we're not careful.

Fortunately for you, I'm going to systematically and thoroughly destroy any argument this voice in your head might have, so we can stop focusing on what's impossible and shift the focus away from, "I can't, because" and toward "Okay, this is my current situation, let's fix it."

Let the great court case of "Inner Voice of Excuses versus *Level Up Your Life*" commence!

EXCUSE #1: BUT I DON'T HAVE TIME

The most common excuse I hear every day as to why people can't level up their lives is: "I just don't have enough time." We've all said it before, and it's probably the loudest argument that voice in our head will make while you're reading this book. We say, "I don't have time" when life gets busy or when we don't want to feel guilty about skipping something:

- ✳ If we don't have enough time to exercise, it's easier for us to be okay with wheezing after climbing a flight of stairs.
- ✳ If we don't have time to apply for new jobs and make new connections, it's easier to accept staying in a job we despise.
- ✳ If we don't have time to work daily on learning a new language, it makes it easier for us to say, "I'll learn it eventually."

Starting today, that voice in your head is no longer allowed to utter the words: "I don't have time." Instead, the voice must use the phrase, "It's not a priority." Watch how quickly your perspective shifts when looking at life's challenges this way:

- ✳ "I'd love to exercise, but I just don't have time" becomes "exercising isn't a priority."
- ✳ "I'd love to learn a new language, but I don't have time to practice" becomes "learning a new language isn't a priority."
- ✳ "I don't have time to find a new job" becomes "finding a new job isn't a priority."

Suddenly, the excuse of having no time gets redefined as "not a priority." I learned this tactic from Laura Vanderkam in her *Wall*

Street Journal article "Are You as Busy as You Think?" and it radically changed how I spend my free time.

I can see that voice in your head fighting back: "Steve, these things ARE a priority, but there just aren't enough hours in the day." As J.D. Roth, creator of GetRichSlowly.org, explained in a keynote speech at the World Domination Summit (a conference in Portland, Oregon): "It's not what we say is a priority, but what we actually do that's a priority."

J.D. shared how he used to tell his friends, "Oh I LOVE reading, I just don't have time for it." In reality, J.D. was just putting everything else in front of reading: watching TV, staying up late surfing the Interwebs, and so on. Once he realized how he was prioritizing his life, he started analyzing where his precious time was going. We have 168 hours in a week, and time is our most precious resource. How are you spending your time? Your priorities, whether you say so or not, are where you choose to spend those hours. It's not what you say that's important to you, it's what you DO that's important to you.

Of course, if you're a single mom working three jobs and have two kids, then I get it: taking care of those kids and putting food on the table understandably must be prioritized over most things. In this situation, we can accept the fact that the Game of Life is being played on Legendary difficulty and you can try to find opportunities to work on the things that will improve your situation whenever and wherever you can. That being said, The Rebellion does include a number of single parents who are finding adventure in their lives, too, so don't be afraid to look to them for inspiration and advice!

So, I challenge the voice in your head, starting today, to erase the phrase "I don't have time" from its vocabulary. Instead, your voice must say, "It's not a priority." If you're truly committed to building your life into something you're proud of, then that has to take priority over Facebook, over video games, over watching cat videos on YouTube, over TV, and so on. Once we stop allowing ourselves to say, "I don't have time," and truly look at where our time is being spent, we will find some pockets of time here and there for focusing on growth and on the quests and missions we need to complete in order to level up.

EXCUSE #2: I CAN'T AFFORD IT

The tiny voices in our heads that complain about not having enough time are no strangers to the "I can't afford it" argument, either. It's this argument that pollutes our brain into justifying not spending money on what's important. Whether it's going on a trip or taking lessons in a skill you want to learn, when that tiny voice in your head tells you that you "can't afford" a trip or a lesson or a class in a skill you want to learn, you are left with three options:

1. Complain loudly to anybody who will listen;
2. Stop spending money on the unimportant;
3. Find a way to make more money on the side.

I've found the first option doesn't really help anybody, at all, ever. Let's look into options two and three, then. Just as we can look at how our time is spent and say, "It's not what we say that's important, but what we do that's important," a look at our spending history quickly reveals what we've deemed important in our lives. Do you:

* Spend $150 a month on cable TV?
* Go out to a $10 lunch each day and grab takeout food on the way home?
* Buy new clothes/shoes monthly?
* Own a car that's brand new or leased?
* Own a home that's bigger than you need?

In order for us to quiet the "I don't have enough money" critic in our brains, we need to do whatever we can to stop spending money on the unimportant so we can reallocate those financial resources to things that provide us with sustainable happiness. Just as how we spend our time determines our priorities, every dollar spent is a vote for what's important in our lives. What would your monthly credit card bill say about your priorities?

First, we can start by cutting out the stuff that's actually detrimental to our health and happiness. If you find you spend too much time watching TV or playing games, cancel your cable and put off buying any new games for the next few months as you get your life in order. Instead of eating out for every meal, bring your lunch to work a few times a week. Stop going out to movies or spending hundreds of dollars at the bars and instead choose to spend a few extra nights every month at home with friends.

Megan Morgalis is a Rebel and incredible world traveler, having visited five continents and 15 countries in the past few years. She even volunteered multiple times at an orphanage in Peru. She does all of this on a seventh grade teacher's salary. How? She spends deliberately: she rents a room in somebody else's house; she doesn't own a television; she drives a 15-year-old car; she doesn't have a smart phone; she even earns extra money by working a side job; and saves every penny she can.

Megan has prioritized adventure and travel, cutting ruthlessly from spending money on things that aren't important to her so she can spend money on things that *are* important: flights, trips, and adventures. Not coincidentally, Megan is the quite possibly the happiest and most content person I have ever met.

The Game of Life doesn't need to be expensive! From learning to speak a new language for free, to sleeping on fellow adventurer's couches, to travel hacking your flights so you can travel cheaply, I guarantee the amount of money required to pull off your dream Game of Life is much smaller than you think. Remember my James Bond story from the Introduction? I MADE money that weekend, including all flights, hotel, tux, and entertainment. The tux rental was only $60. I used hotel points thanks to some crafty travel hacking, so the room was free. And I actually won a few hundred bucks at the blackjack table!

If you have more disposable income, then this might be less of an issue for you, but you can still find plenty of opportunities to have adventures and learn new skills without spending a dime or even leaving your hometown. You often simply need to redefine your vision of how a certain adventure might play out—doing it on the cheap is more adventurous anyway!

EXCUSE #3: BUT MY JOB WON'T ALLOW IT

Ah yes, your job. The way you make a living, and the way you pay for all of the awesomeness listed above. A recent *Forbes* article pointed out a Gallup poll that showed "unhappy employees outnumber happy ones by two to one" worldwide. This means most people are either in a role that doesn't align with their strengths or they have no opportunities to grow and advance within their companies. I was fortunate enough to be so unhappy with my day job that I needed to make a drastic change, but most people are merely a bit dissatisfied with their jobs and thus never make a change that allows them to live out the adventurous life of a hero.

Here's the truth: life is freaking short, and tomorrow isn't guaranteed. On top of that, we spend a majority of our waking hours at our jobs. And we know that the number one regret of dying people is that they hadn't lived true to themselves. So where does that leave us?

Ultimately, reality tells us that we're expected to bust our asses in jobs we don't like, getting stressed out on a day-to-day basis, cramming our vacations into a few long weekends a year (if we can get over the guilt we feel when we actually take vacations), and then we get so stressed out about the work we did or the work we have to do when we get back that we barely enjoy the vacation itself!

The great news about working in a job that leaves you unfulfilled and unhappy is that it doesn't need to define you. Until there's an opportunity to make a change, you can put your focus on growing and advancing in your spare time. Or, you can start by making your adventure about breaking free first, before moving on to the next quest. Not only that, but you always have the option to quit. I have a hunch that you're a pretty resourceful person, so why not move onto a friend's couch, sell your car, move to a cheaper state, and give a different path a shot? It certainly beats the alternative of being miserable for 50–80 hours a week for the rest of your life, right?

Please understand that I'm not advising you to quit your job and follow your dreams on a whim. Oftentimes, quitting or changing careers is the right decision, but that depends on your specific situation. Even though I've quit two jobs, I did both with a very good reason and gave myself a solid chance to succeed with the next opportunity. So if there's a way to set up the next experience before quitting your job, I always recommend this path. But there might be an even easier solution: can you have a discussion with your boss about finding ways for you to grow and make more of an impact at your current job?

> SO, RATHER THAN CHASING MORE MONEY, WE INSTEAD SHOULD BE FOCUSING ON WHY WE WANT MORE MONEY. AND FOR MOST OF US, IT'S BECAUSE IT BUYS US FREEDOM.

I understand that we all need to make a living, and that we sometimes feel like our jobs have us on a path that's set in stone. This feeling only grows stronger as we get older. I can promise you that it's never too late to start or make a change or try something new. After I quit my job to build Nerd Fitness, it was pretty neat watching my father retire from a job he held for 30 years to start up his own company, too.

Let's be honest here. The real reason we stay for far longer than we'd like in jobs we don't like is often because of our co-workers, because of the security, or because of the amount of money it provides. Believe it or not, the age-old saying is true: "Money can't buy you happiness." In fact, a 2010 Princeton Study showed that once we make more than a certain amount of money, more of it does not bring more happiness.

So, rather than chasing more money, we instead should be focusing on why we want more money. And for most of us, it's because it buys us freedom.

Freedom to travel.

Freedom to spend more time with friends and family.

Freedom to not have to worry about our monthly mortgage and other bill payments.

Freedom to enjoy the finer things in life.

As we are rearranging our lives around the things that are important to us, we need to understand that our jobs and career paths aren't set in stone; there's nothing other than that tiny voice in our head keeping us from making career happiness a focus.

Make sure you read the Rebel Spotlight in Chapter 4 about Kishi, a man who lived below the poverty line and got his life together to make it to an adventure race with fellow Nerd Fitness Rebels.

EXCUSE #4: BUT I'M TOO OLD

Whoever said, "You can't teach an old dog new tricks" is a liar, liar, pants on fire. Suzanne Collins wrote The Hunger Games at age 46. Tamae Watanabe of Japan summited Mount Everest at the age of 73, 10 years after setting the previous record at 63! Even my dad recently retired from his day job after 30 years at 63 to start his own company. In doing research for this book, I met many Rebels over the age of 70, including Gay from New Mexico who is 73, has nine grandchildren, and lost 90 pounds on her journey!

They may be clichés, but age is only a number, and you're only as old as you feel. Whether you're 20 or 50 or 80, there's nothing other than that voice in your head to stop you from making positive changes in your life and focusing on building a game that makes you happy, regardless of your age. When 2014 Boston Marathon champion Meb Keflezighi was asked how long he thought he could continue competing at an elite level, now being over the age of 40, he responded: "If no one ever told you when you were born, how would you know how old you are?"

Here's my favorite quote from *The Shawshank Redemption*: "Get busy livin', or get busy dyin'." I actually have a pillow on my couch with this printed on it to remind me every day that I have this choice. So ask yourself: Can I find a way to be happier and healthier today than I was yesterday? Can I find a way to make life more fulfilling today than it was at this time last year? It's never too late to change, you're never too old to learn, and you're never too far down a path to change to a different one. As humans, we have the amazing ability to change and adapt code into our DNA.

EXCUSE #5: BUT I DON'T HAVE THE SAME OPPORTUNITIES AS OTHER PEOPLE

This might be my favorite argument, because it's something we all do. We see the opportunities or success other people have had and instead of asking "How can I do that?" or "Where can I get started?" the voice in our head says things like "Must be nice, but . . ." or "If only I had [insert some random opportunity], then I could succeed." I get a few emails a week from people who tell me I'm lucky, and that they could never do what I've done. I'm just a normal guy who had access to the Internet and a desire to better himself. Yes, I realize that I'm fortunate to have grown up with loving parents who have been supportive of my decisions, but I know of many members of The Rebellion who had to go it alone and struggled with a less than optimal upbringing. A quick look at the Rebel Spotlights throughout this book will reveal people from all walks of life leveling up. My initial investment to start Nerd Fitness was $100 to buy a domain and web hosting. I have a hunch that if you're reading this book, then you, too, have access to the Internet and a desire to live a better, happier life. No matter where you come from or where you are now, today represents an opportunity to be better than you were yesterday.

We all have to play life on different difficulty levels. Some people are born with superior genetics, or to rich parents, and never have to work a day in their lives: these people are playing the game on Easy mode (and they might struggle with finding true meaning!). Others are born into broken homes, in third-world countries, with chronic ailments or into poor school systems, and they have to play the game on Legendary difficulty. The greater the origin story, the more dramatic the Hero's Journey. We can either complain about the character we've rolled, or we can acknowledge it and then play that character to the best of our ability.

It's often not our fault for the situation or place in life we're in, but it is our responsibility to try to fix it. Once we accept that, understanding that nobody else is going to dig us out of the hole, we become empowered. We give ourselves permission to change our path, to alter our destiny, to change our fate.

So, we need to tell the voice in our head that keeps saying, "Well, I can't do this because . . ." to be quiet. We all have baggage, and we all have things we're working through. We all have obligations, and we all have things about ourselves that we don't like. Putting all of that aside, we all share one thing that is going to give us a leg up: a genuine desire for a better life and, with this book, the knowledge to make it happen.

EXCUSE #6: LIFE ISN'T A FAIRY TALE, MOVIE, OR GAME. BE REALISTIC.

When we look at our existence as something that must be endured, every challenge reinforces our negative attitude, and we end up miserable. When we look at life through the lens of a Hero's Journey, every challenge becomes an opportunity to learn and grow and emerge transformed.

We only get a few brief years on this planet, and members of The Rebellion have chosen to live those years as if they are characters playing a role in an epic story—and why the hell not! Life is supposed to be fun, and when you feel like you are having fun, more good things happen and there's more of an opportunity to live a leveled-up life.

Whether you live for another few days or for another 10 decades, I want you to live a life you can be proud of. I want you to look in the mirror with pride each day, and I want you to look back at the end of your life and say, "Yup, I played this game right."

No more excuses. Instead of coming up with reasons why we can't do the stuff we talk about in this book, we instead must ask, "Okay, what do I need to do, and how do I need to do it in order to make these things a reality?" Now that we've quieted our inner voices and enemies, giving us a chance to get started on our adventure, we need to watch out for the external threats we'll face as well.

And to do that, we're going into the Matrix.

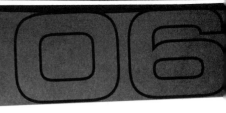

BEWARE DARK FORCES, HIDDEN FOES, AND HATERS

NEO: WHY DO MY EYES HURT?

MORPHEUS: BECAUSE YOU'VE NEVER USED THEM BEFORE.

—THE MATRIX

"Welcome, to the real world."

I'll never forget that jaw-dropping scene from *The Matrix* in which the story's hero, Neo, learns what the Matrix is. He wakes up in the real world and discovers he's been living his entire life inside a computer program designed to keep him prisoner. Although the movie is now well over a decade old, I still think daily about my own life in the Matrix and how I can help others break free from it. Most of us are trapped in it without our knowledge: we've all been programmed to follow a specific set of rules that govern how we exist. For the past 80-plus years, that's gone something like this: get a job for the most money you can, buy the biggest house you can, the nicest car, the biggest television, and work your ass off for 40-plus years until you retire at 65 to finally enjoy the good life. This is the wool that has been pulled over our eyes to keep us complacent and subdued. We're taught and told by everybody around us that this is just the way things are, and we're supposed to follow along and not cause any trouble.

However, just as Neo sat at his computer every night because he knew something was missing, you are reading this book because you, too, know something is missing and you want to find out what it is. Your current situation in life is a result of the role you've played up to this point in the Matrix that is built around you. Happy or sad, good or bad, it's the acceptance of our roles in this system that got us where we are. When things don't go well for us, or we wonder why things aren't better than they are, we usually seek temporary solutions to treat the symptoms rather than addressing the real problem at its source.

INSTEAD OF ASKING, "WHEN DOES LIFE GET FUN AGAIN?" WE'VE REPRIORITIZED WHAT'S IMPORTANT TO US AND ASK: "HOW CAN I HAVE FUN AND GROW TODAY?" WE HAVE OUR ALTER EGOS FOCUSED ON MAKING THOSE THINGS THE PRIORITY, AND THEN WE BUILD THE REST OF THE MATRIX AROUND THOSE THINGS.

Here's an example that is all too common in this day and age: If you come home stressed out from a mentally or physically taxing day, drown your sorrows in a bottle on the couch while playing a game, and then wake up to an alarm clock and chug a pot of coffee to get through the next day, you are trying to operate within a system that is broken and which doesn't work for you. In this particular instance, you're using temporary hacks to treat real, permanent problems: the alcohol to forget the work day, the games to escape a stressful week, and the alarm clock and caffeine to recover from a hangover and sleep deprivation. This is no way to live, and you need to fix it.

Looking at each of your problems individually and trying to patch them to make yourself a little bit happier (if only temporarily) is the equivalent of trying to live properly within the Matrix. However, looking at that entire sequence from a different perspective, we can see we are dealing within a system that needs a major code rewrite at the base level! Instead of patching each of the code's faults as they pop up, we should be instead looking at the source code from the ground up and fixing it so these problems are no longer an issue.

This is why you're joining The Rebellion, a group of like-minded, unlikely heroes who have refused to play nice in the Matrix. Within our movement, we've decided that instead of asking, "When does life get fun again?" we've reprioritized what's important to us and ask: "How can I have fun and grow today?" We have our alter egos focused on making those things the priority, and then we build the rest of the Matrix around those things. As Morpheus tells Neo: "Some rules can be bent, others can be broken." Why not build our lives around the things that truly matter?

You don't need to live the life expected of you. You don't need to be doing something simply because it's always been done that way. And there's nothing telling you that you need to follow the traditional path of the trapped Matrix prisoner: wake up, go to a job, eat, come home, watch TV, sleep, repeat. You might be single and 20, or married and 40, or divorced with three kids at 60. Either way, The Rebellion needs you. Regardless of your current situation, we can get started living a better, healthier, happier life today. Remember Rule #1 of The Rebellion: "We don't care where you came from, only where you're going."

When you can find that happy medium between enjoying today, making improvements, and planning for tomorrow, amazing things start to happen and life gets epic—the story arcs you live start to build on top of each other; each completion of the circle brings more adventure, more stories, more growth, and more personal transformation. Whether you plan on improving your life through a renewed focus on making an impact at work, finding happiness with activities after work, a physical transformation that enables you to participate in more activities, or a focus on travel by radically adjusting how you make a living— changes to the source code will have you seeing ones and zeroes like Neo and have you playing on a completely different level than everybody else around you.

Now, I do have to warn you: as you are starting to reengineer your life around what makes you happy and what best sets you up to achieve heroic success, you're likely going to run into a few types of people who will challenge you and present hurdles. When you decide you no longer want to play by the rules of the Matrix and instead play by your own rules, some will get confused and others might not like it very much. Those still trapped will see you forging your own path and potentially get jealous or tell you to "be realistic." Just as every story has heroes and villains, allies and enemies, so too will your path to success. So that we'll be prepared to defeat them when they inevitably materialize, let's now identify those who might seek to stand in your way:

AGENTS (A.K.A. GUARDIANS)

Think of Agent Smith in *The Matrix*, a piece of the code designed to destroy any and all anomalies. These are the gatekeepers who will try to keep you from living the life you want, keep you from crossing the threshold into your adventurous life, and who don't want you rearranging the code of the Matrix. They've grown comfortable with things just how they are, and they don't want people like you messing it up! The Agent could be a boss who doesn't want you to take your vacation, who wonders why you aren't working nights and weekends, too, and who doesn't value you as an employee. The Agent might be a relationship you're in that has run its course, and the other person in it is afraid you're going to leave them behind when you level up your life and make positive changes.

Agents don't want you to break free or become the hero you're on the path to become, and will do anything to keep you locked up as a prisoner in their program. Depending on how involved these people are with your life, they can present a very real and serious challenge to your future as a Rebel.

PEOPLE WHO HAVEN'T BROKEN FREE YET

When you decide to start living life on your terms with a priority on adventure, those who are still blissfully unaware of their existence in the Matrix might give you funny looks when you start talking about the growth and adventures you envision for yourself. They are still caught up in the Matrix and are either uninterested in breaking out or unaware they can break free. I got plenty of weird looks and comments from people who were confused when I told them that, at age 30, I decided I wanted to learn to play the violin. These people could be your friends and family members. They'll tell you that you're crazy, that you should be reasonable, that you should be more realistic with your goals and expectations. It could also be colleagues, or classmates, or random strangers on the Internet telling you how to live your life.

Author Seth Godin put it plainly: "Be judged, or be ignored." If you want to do extraordinary things, and you plan on standing out from the crowd, expect to be judged for it. Perhaps harshly. After initially being bothered by this judgment, I started wearing it like a badge of honor. I remember everybody thinking I was nuts when I told them I planned on quitting my job to move across the country to take a job for a 50 percent pay cut. Then everybody thought I was completely insane when I eventually quit a dream job to start my own company and focus on adventure. I was very fortunate to have a really supportive family that knew I'd find a way to make things work, but I know many people who had to go it alone when they chose to prioritize adventure. If I'm going to be labeled a weirdo for wanting to improve my life and do really fun things, I'm okay with that. Fortunately, we now have an actual group of Rebels who refuse to accept mediocrity and can offer up support and encouragement along the way.

On top of that, we all become freed from the Matrix at different times, and we can be there for these people in our lives when they're ready to follow a heroic path, too.

How you choose to break free from these Agents and deal with those who haven't broken free yet is up to you and your tolerance for change. What I am saying is that when you try to break free from the Matrix and reprioritize your life around adventure, growth, and happiness, you're most likely going to get pushback from those around you, and it's to be expected.

HATERS GONNA HATE

If you've spent any time on Xbox Live, then you've encountered "the hater." It's usually a 12-year-old male who spends his time on Xbox yelling racial, sexist, and/or homophobic slurs at anybody who happens to beat him in a battle. Heck, you might have even BEEN that 12-year old back in the day.

When we encounter haters in a game, we quickly brush them off and say, "They have no idea what they're talking about." We can ban them or block them or report them—and we know we never, in fact, had relations with a member of the equine family.

However, how are we supposed to behave when we encounter haters in real life? If you are on the path to a better life, whether it's starting your own business, traveling to a foreign country, or even trying to get healthy, you're going to encounter haters at every turn. These people have the uncanny ability to take any situation and find a way to say something negative about it:

* I'm traveling to a foreign country: "Why would you want to go there? I hear it's dangerous. Not me, thanks."
* I'm building a business: "You're crazy! You already have a good job. Why would you want to do something so risky?"
* I'm learning to play the piano: "Ha! Good luck. I know somebody who has been playing for years, so you're gonna be awful for a long time. Why even bother?"

These people will find a way to rain on any parade, and the more you try to change and improve yourself, the more they'll push back with reasons why it won't work.

The truth is that most people fear change. They, themselves, might want to change but don't want to put forth the effort and energy to make it happen. Or perhaps seeing somebody else making positive changes makes them feel insecure about their own situation, so they choose instead to try to drag you back down. Despite the fact that I run a positive business that focuses on encouraging people to find happiness, I've had some amazing insults publicly thrown in my direction—venomous things that nobody would dare say to my face. But that's life for a Rebel. It's important to remember that most people who are insulting or angry are really just struggling with unhappiness or dissatisfaction in their own lives and need somebody to take it out on.

When I tell people that I traveled the world and came back more financially stable than when I left, I can't tell you how many times I heard, "Must be nice to be young and blah blah blah like you Steve . . . I can't do that because [insert excuse here]." I know single moms who have taken adventurous trips with their kids, broke couples who traveled and have continued to do so, and elderly folks who decided, "Why not today? I'm not getting any younger," and set off on an adventure. But haters don't want to hear that! They'd much rather sit back and make excuses for why they can't do things that would make them happy instead of taking a chance or putting in the work. Oh well!

When I quit my day job to focus on helping people get healthy with Nerd Fitness, I ignored those who told me I was nuts and busted my ass for years to make sure I stayed afloat until the business took off. Everybody has an opinion, and when you decide to do something different than what the masses are doing, haters won't hesitate to tell you about it.

HOW TO DEAL WITH HATERS

I remember the first negative comment I ever got on Nerd Fitness. This random dude decided to go off on me with a comment full of hatred and factual inaccuracies. Naïve and hurt, I decided it was my responsibility to help teach this anonymous Internet person that he was wrong. I spent three hours crafting a response with citations and sources explaining my side and sent it to him. He came back with, "You actually read what I wrote? I was just having a bad day and needed to vent. Whatever."

I had spent three hours of my existence trying to win over a guy who had no desire to be won over. And since my site has grown, so too has the target on my back. Now the attacks are even more brutal, personal, and frequent. But I ignore them and move on with my life! Spending any time thinking about haters is a waste of energy, as that's time that could be spent helping more people or working to improve yourself. Life is too damn short to give any power to these non-contributing zeros, so I do the real-life equivalent of "block" when it's somebody who isn't part of my life.

But what can you do if a hater happens to be one of your friends or loved ones? If you are trying to do something positive or healthy with your life, it can be quite difficult when you are surrounded by friends who are not interested in improving their own lives but have no problem telling you how to live yours. You're so excited to tell them about your new deadlift record or to invite them on a cave expedition, but all they want to do is game or drink and make fun of you for being healthy and skipping Taco Tuesday.

HATERS
GONNA HATE

These comments serve a singular purpose—to make haters, even if they are friends of yours, feel better about themselves. It's not that these people truly want to put you down or see you fail, but these remarks take way less effort (and are much less scary) than if they actually tried to change themselves. They might be afraid of trying to change their lives and failing, or maybe they have already tried and failed, and see your success as validation of that failure.

We all have these negative people in our lives, and it can truly be depressing. It feels like we're a mutant who hasn't found the X-Men Academy yet; we feel like the only person in our group who wants to "evolve" and therefore must deal with being an outcast. Sure, The Rebellion can be your online support community, but what about those people who tell you to your face that you're going to fail or that you shouldn't bother trying?

Some people are just unhappy at the moment (like that random Internet dude), and other people just aren't ready to change yet. Many people will hate on the success and positive change of those around them because those things make them feel worse about themselves. Just remember, it's not about you, but about them. And you don't have to accept it.

Here is your four-step plan for dealing with haters:

1. **Understand that judgment is inevitable.** We all get judged every minute of every day, no matter what we do (or don't). I've officially adopted the stance that if I'm going to get judged for something, being judged for being healthy, nerding out about interesting topics, and going on adventures is a pretty damn good thing! This required a mental shift for me to realize that it's a badge of honor to be considered "the weird one."

2. **Consider the source.** Constructive criticism can be an important part of growth and change, but it's also very important to consider the source of the criticism. If you are getting criticized for your new lifestyle by somebody who is out of shape, unhappy, overweight, and generally miserable, it's probably not worth your time and effort to worry about it! I often just smile and nod (while being proud on the inside), or just say, "Ha ha, I know, I'm weird, right?"

3. **Get them on board.** Many accidental haters (usually family members) don't realize the damage their comments/remarks are doing to your efforts to improve yourself. Part of the Hero's Journey can often be about outsmarting or enlisting/ changing the guardian of the threshold to the Hero's Cause. Consider this part of your test! Explain to them that you're trying to change and that you want their support and help. Tell them you're trying to win a contest at work, or that you have a personal challenge you're trying to complete, and that you want to see if you can actually follow through with it.

   These otherwise well-meaning detractors can become

your biggest supporters if you ask for their help—everybody wants to feel like they're making a difference, right? And who knows, you might inspire them with your actions.

4. **Consider how you spend your most valuable asset: time.** As I've heard consistently and truly believe, you become the average of the five people you associate most with. If you are spending your time with "Negative Nancies" and haters who are not taking steps to better their lives, it probably feels like you are running through quicksand while trying to build momentum. Instead of surrounding yourself with people who are dragging you down, why not surround yourself with people who elevate and pull you up? We'll discuss this in greater detail in Chapter 16.

Now that we've established that we don't have to accept life in the Matrix, or the opinions of haters or other negative forces, we're going to dig deep and get to the source of what we want to accomplish in our Game of Life. We're going to take steps, every single day, toward realizing our goals. We're going to learn how to stop relying on motivation and willpower, how to make procrastination a thing of the past and, instead, build a set of game rules and hacks for the Matrix that's custom-built for our success.

Remember, we need to build our life around the adventures we want to live and the things we want to learn about. That way, the adventures and growth that result from them become our priority.

Just as the Matrix was a challenge for Neo, our journey will be a challenge as well—fortunately, life is a multiplayer game, and all stories have many characters. I just taught you how to deal with haters along your journey. Later on, I'll cover how to surround yourself with an amazing fellowship to help you succeed. And by prioritizing a life focused on helping us to become the best versions of ourselves, we also, in turn, prioritize the truest goals of our existence as humans: freedom and happiness.

07

EMBRACE GAMIFICATION TO UNLOCK HAPPINESS

IT'S DANGEROUS TO GO ALONE! TAKE THIS.

—*THE OLD MAN*, THE LEGEND OF ZELDA

Believe it or not, hidden within our favorite video games are the secrets to our happiness. From Zelda to Mario, Call of Duty to *World of Warcraft*, video games have discovered the fundamental principles that can teach us how to live better, happier lives. After all, there's a reason why this book is called *Level Up Your Life.* I'm talking about happiness in real life! At some point in our lives, we've all said one of the following:

* ✳ "If I just had more money, I'd be happy."

* ✳ "If I just had a bigger TV/car/house, I'd be happy."

* ✳ "If I just looked more like that guy/girl, I'd be happy."

* ✳ "If I just got that promotion, I'd be happy."

And there's nothing inherently wrong with these thoughts—having goals is incredibly important in this nerd's opinion—except that if we're not careful, they can cause us to head down a path we're not so thrilled to be on. We often tie our happiness to getting the things we desire. Certainly, ambition is important, but are we deluding ourselves by interlocking the two? While we are building our new existence as an adventurous alter ego, we too often assume we need things we don't have in order to be successful. It turns out that it's actually the pursuit of these things and the challenges we encounter along the way that fuel our happiness, not the items themselves. Once we earn beyond a certain amount of money, more of it won't necessarily make us happier—there are many other daily things that drastically impact how we feel each and every day.

DISCOVERING HAPPINESS AT AGE FIVE

Ever since I was a little kid, I've been in love with the idea of leveling up. I remember playing the *Legend of Zelda* for the Nintendo Entertainment System (NES), wandering into that mysterious cave on the opening screen, taking the wooden sword from the weird old dude, and setting out to save the land of Hyrule. Link was just this little kid, scared out of his mind, working hard to get stronger and fight bigger bad guys until he could save Zelda. I immediately related: I was a small guy, also scared out of my mind of pretty much everything, so I felt like I could be Link. In fact, I remember one time making a bow and arrow in my backyard while pretending I WAS Link. Unfortunately, I accidentally used leaves from a poison ivy plant to make the "feathers" on my arrows, which resulted in a swollen face and hand for about a week. Oops.

As I grew older, I moved on to more complex role-playing games that still had a strong focus on leveling systems and progressions. The graphics improved, the stories got better, and the level of immersion got me more hooked than ever before. Once I rebuilt my life around adventure rather than escape, I studied the exact mechanics used to capture the hearts and minds of gamers like myself throughout the world. I figured if they could keep us glued to our computer chairs and couches instead of being outside, interacting with the real world, there had to be a way to learn from them to improve our lives beyond the screen. And, thus, I've devoted a significant portion of my time trying to figure out what makes video games so addicting.

I loved the Legend of Zelda series because there was always something to find, a new place to discover, a new secret to uncover beneath a burned bush or behind a false wall, a new dungeon to crawl through.

I loved *EverQuest* and *EverQuest 2* because I got to play as the powerful, erudite wizard, Morphos Novastorm. Wizards always start out as the weakest characters in RPGs, underpowered and vulnerable, but by the time one reaches the end of the game, they are the most powerful.

I loved *Assassin's Creed II* (and its direct sequels) because I wanted to become Ezio Auditore da Firenze, a member of the Assassin order during the Italian Renaissance: constantly earning better weapons, exploring new locations, performing parkour, scaling massive ruins, and taking part in grand historical fiction.

I combined all of these things and decided to put their greatest strengths to the test in the real world. My discovery was pretty freaking awesome. After analyzing them, it became clear to me that these games, along with hundreds of others that have captivated the attention of nerds over the years, not only provide us with entertainment, but with exact instructions for how to manufacture lasting happiness as a priority in our lives. Just as the characters followed a Hero's Journey, so too could we be on our path to happiness and transformation.

Here's how.

THE GAME MECHANICS
OF HAPPINESS

Nerds tend to have very addictive personalities, and video games have been designed to push every one of our "this makes me happy" buttons to keep us blissfully addicted. It turns out that, once we understand how our brains work and apply a bit of behavioral psychology to our understanding of the games we love to play, we can ourselves become characters in these games, capable of leveling up, too. These sources for escape and entertainment can be some of the best motivational tools at our disposal if we look at them with the correct mindset. So, let's look at the mechanics that keeps gamers coming back for more and more and more.

GAMES AND STORIES ALLOW US TO LIVE OUT EPIC EXISTENCES

Whether we are saving the princess, traveling to Mordor to destroy the One Ring, or exploring far-off locales like Lara Croft in *Tomb Raider*, these games and stories give us a chance to escape boring lives and instead imagine life as the hero. It's tough to do that in real life when we never go anywhere other than to our home or office. It's also tough if we are out of shape and physically unable to do many of the things the character in the game or story can do.

GAMES HAVE A VERY SPECIFIC LEVELING SYSTEM

When you are Level 1 and killing spiders, you know that when you kill enough spiders, you get to level up eventually and get to start attacking rats. Once you advance to a high enough level, you know you get to start slaying FREAKING DRAGONS (which can only be written in all caps). Because there is a very clearly defined path for you to follow, it's easy to know what you have to do next or what you get to do next, and thus it's as simple as killing enough bad guys, or completing enough quests, and so on. The path from Zero to Hero is clearly defined.

GAMES HAVE A REWARD SYSTEM

When you reach Level 5 in *EverQuest* or *World of Warcraft*, you might earn a new sword that will make getting to Level 6 easier, which then gets you a better spell that allows you to kill bad guys even faster. This system of dangling that carrot in front of you is a powerful force in pushing gamers to say, "Just five more minutes." We've all been there, spending far too many hours late into the night chasing "just one more quest." This reward system is instant, gratifying, and incredibly satisfying. The greater the challenge, the bigger the quest, the more satisfying the reward. If you've ever seen any of those studies in which rats press a button and then are rewarded with cheese, you understand that a cue and reward can be incredibly powerful.

GAMES ENCOURAGE EXPLORATION

In most RPGs there's always something new to explore or accomplish that keeps you guessing and looking forward to whatever's next. You might wonder what's over that mountain range, or at the bottom of that lake, or in that cave, or what the next zone will be. This one element alone is enough for me to stay up far too late playing a game and exploring.

GAMES GIVE US A CHANCE TO ACHIEVE "FLOW" AND MASTERY

Ever heard of video game speed runs? Or seen the documentary *The King of Kong*? Watched somebody just dominate a game of *Tetris*? Games are an opportunity for us to get lost in the flow of a game, to zone out while perfecting our skills and seeing if we can complete a particular section or level faster, more efficiently, and/or with more points. I've probably completed *Metroid Prime* for the GameCube a dozen times, each time working on finding new pathways, new secrets, and hacks to bypass entire sections, in a quest to complete the game in under two hours (Now it turns out there are people who have completed it in only an hour!). There's actually a scientific term for what happens when we enter this trancelike state while playing a game, and we'll explain why getting into this state can change your life. Watching people at the peak of a particular game's skill level is a sight to behold (just

Google "Speed Run + [your favorite game]" and enjoy).

These are the reasons why I've been addicted to any particular game at one point or another, and I'm sure you can probably relate. They happen to hit all of the right buttons and switches and nerves in my brain that make me want to play more. In fact, I was supposed to be working on this book recently, but instead jumped into a game of *Diablo III* with my friends for a few hours, even though I've already beaten it a few times. Thinking back, I realize it's because the game possessed all of the mechanics I highlighted earlier: I could zone out and get lost in the flow of kicking ass, connect with friends, challenge increasingly more difficult bad guys, collect new armor, and level up my character.

It's time to identify how we can do those things in real life, and then actually get started with doing them!

HAPPINESS IN A NUTSHELL: GROW AND FLOW

We can boil down what we do every day as humans and what we hope to accomplish in our lives to a single goal: the realization of happiness. As Sigmund Freud pointed out, at our most basic level we seek to avoid pain and gain pleasure. Believe it or not, we can use research-backed studies and science to help us be happier, and we can use the very games we previously highlighted to make it happen.

For starters, we are happy when we are making progress. If you've ever spent hours killing the same bad guys repeatedly to level up in a video game, this will not come as a surprise to you. We love making progress so much that we actually enjoy it more than getting the thing we wanted in the first place! It doesn't need to be big progress, just enough that we realize we are moving forward, improving, getting better. Incremental improvement can actually be addictive. These short-term wins release dopamine—the happiness chemical—in our brains, and we crave more. This is referred to as the "Progress Principle." Just like in games, if we can find a way to make small improvements and recognize those small improvements in our day-to-day lives, it's likely to increase our overall happiness. Again, it doesn't matter what our starting point is or how wealthy or successful we are currently, only that we are progressing and improving day after day.

The "Adaptation Level Principle" helps us understand this phenomenon. Researchers at the University of California, Santa Barbara, looked at two groups of people: those who had just won the lottery and those who had recently become paraplegics. Initially and unsurprisingly, the lottery winners experienced extremely high happiness and the paraplegic group was simply devastated. But one year later both groups were more or less equally happy. More than that, the paraplegics reported being happier in accomplishing everyday tasks than the lottery winners were. Thus, the happiness we achieve by chasing bigger, better, newer, or shinier rewards quickly fades. Our new "happy" quickly becomes our new "normal," causing us to chase even bigger and better rewards to fill our happiness void! In other words, trying to tie our happiness to shinier and shinier objects isn't sustainable— it's incremental progress that creates long-term, lasting happiness.

So, as we start to develop the life we want to live, we're going to keep this philosophy at the front of our minds—we need to make progress and show ourselves that we are making progress. Let me give you a few key examples:

Workers who are expanding their skill sets and who are regularly able to find solutions to day-to-day challenges are far happier and productive than people who don't. As Harvard Business School professor Teresa Amabile demonstrates in her TEDx talk about the "Progress Principle," ensuring that employees are improving is absolutely essential to keeping morale and productivity high. When you feel like you are stuck at status quo, happiness and performance plummet.

If you're unhappy in your job, is it because there's no room to grow, to progress, to learn new skills and advance? Do you feel like you aren't learning anything new at school in your classes or studies? If adjustments within your current job—or a change of professions— isn't an option right now, I'd bet a Master Sword that picking a new skill you enjoy and working to improve it in your spare time will make you happier. Fortunately, there are resources available to you through which you can learn new skills and work on them daily for free or for a nominal cost, for example: Treehouse.com, KhanAcademy.org, and CodeAcademy.com. Feeling like you are progressing and learning while at school or work is a huge part of what keeps us happy and motivated, so if that's not possible as part of your day job, you can focus on adding it into your alter ego's after-work existence.

Joe Rougeux has been a member of The Rebellion since the first day it existed, for he was my college roommate and we've been friends ever since! I remember watching Joe spend hours every day in college working his way up to number one in the world on *Halo 2* on Xbox Live, hilariously singing *The Lion King*'s "I Just Can't Wait to be King" as he destroyed the competition. After college, Joe went to work as a programmer for a company that wasn't aligned with his strengths. It paid well, but he knew something was missing but couldn't quite put his finger on it. After a few years of existing, Joe stumbled across a job post looking for a developer at Hi-Rez Studios, the video game company behind *Tribes Ascend* and *Smite!* There was only one prob-

> JUST LIKE IN GAMES, IF WE CAN FIND A WAY TO MAKE SMALL IMPROVEMENTS AND RECOGNIZE THOSE SMALL IMPROVEMENTS IN OUR DAY-TO-DAY LIVES, IT'S LIKELY TO INCREASE OUR OVERALL HAPPINESS.

lem: Joe had never programmed a game in his life! So he devoted all of his free time to learning to code in the Unreal Engine, applied for the job, and then kicked everybody's ass in the first-person shooter game the company was developing. Joe was hired shortly thereafter, and thanks to loving his job so much he quickly worked his way onwards and upwards. The company gave Joe freedom to experiment, grow and learn, and try new things. He's now one of the lead developers on Hi-Rez's next major project. It's been

CONTINUED ON PAGE 72

REBEL HERO

★ ★ ★ ★ ★ ★

NAME: Ian O'Beirne   **AGE:** 29

HOMETOWN: Pennsauken, NJ

The first thing I did after joining The Rebellion was to re-title my "Tasks" list "Quests." This simple change has spread profoundly into the rest of my life as a keystone habit.

This led to another quest, starting a bullet journal and going fully analog with my quest list, and I've fully decked it out as a monthly list of goals titled "Adventures."

In my life as a full-time touring musician, I've seen the lower 48, Canada, Japan, and Portugal. For the first few years, I fell into the pattern of drinking constantly, becoming angry and complaining about the other musicians, focusing on the negative and thinking about making yet another change instead of sticking something out.

Then The Rebellion came along and changed my perspective on everything. I learned from it that perspective is where everything begins, and by changing my lifestyle and habits, I've changed my perspective in fundamental ways. I get to do what I love and I treat every gig and even every long travel day like a boss battle.

Paradoxically, this focus on accomplishing quests has allowed me to live more in the moment, maintain consistency in practicing my music and living a lifestyle of fitness. My habits have changed and I'll choose the salad instead of the fries without even really thinking about it. It is easy to become

SPOTLIGHT

DAY JOB: *Touring Jazz Musician*

ALTER EGO: *Slowburn*　　　　**CLASS:** *Troubador*

lazy, dark, and alcoholic when work separates you from your family and friends, but The Rebellion has allowed me to swim upstream and jump over the biggest rocks in the way in order to structure my life into something meaningful.

Now I'm even playing the bassoon and making my own reeds!! Every other woodwind doubler tells me I'm crazy for doing it, but I'm no longer even paying attention to the naysayers and just doing everything that once seemed impossible. Even when life gets rocky, which it does, I still look forward to opening my adventure log and tackling the challenges that crop up.

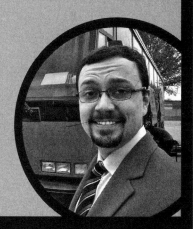

> THE GOAL IS TO PRESENT YOURSELF WITH CHALLENGES YOU ARE CAPABLE OF OVERCOMING, BUT WHICH ARE STILL CHALLENGING ENOUGH TO ENGAGE ALL OF YOUR ATTENTION.

a blast watching Joe level up his life and I couldn't be happier that he has found what he is meant to do. Not coincidentally, Joe has never been happier.

Along with being able to get hooked on making progress with healthy aspects in our lives, happiness is also strongly correlated with us getting into "the zone." As Jonathan Haidt describes in his book, *The Happiness Hypothesis*, we have a basic need to make things happen. Haidt explains how Harry Harlow, a famous psychologist who studied rhesus monkeys, once took his students to the zoo. They unexpectedly found that the monkeys solved problems simply for fun. At the time this confused behaviorists, since they believed that all animals only reacted to positive or negative reinforcements: a prize for doing something good, or punishment for doing something bad. But it turns out this drive to solve problems is innate in us.

As children we seek out toys to learn more about our world, to solve simple problems and engage with our environment. As adults we love to feel productive, and similarly feel a void when we sit around doing nothing. Haidt defines being productive and happy as "flow," a concept coined by psychology professor Mihály Csíkszentmihályi. Haidt explains it as "the mental state of operation in which a person performing an activity is fully immersed in a feeling of energized focus, full involvement, and enjoyment in the process of the activity."

What tasks, hobbies, or jobs can you recall in which you lost track of time? Was it while playing music? Working on a puzzle or quilt? An intense coding session? Thanks to Albert Einstein, we know time is relative, and that's no more apparent when we are spending time doing things we love. So start thinking about the things that help you lose track of time now, and later in the book we'll put a more concrete plan in place to focus on these things.

If we seek happiness as a daily goal, then we can start by focusing on a career and hobbies that provide us with an opportunity to find progress and flow. Whether it's making progress in a job that excites us instead of the one that pays the most money, a hobby that ignites our passions, and/or a workout or adventure or trip of a lifetime we can immerse ourselves in, we have a chance to finish a day happy because we are doing what we're biologically engineered to do. The goal is to present yourself with challenges you are capable of overcoming, but which are still challenging enough to engage all of your attention. Sound familiar? It's like defeating that last boss of a game that requires insane concentration, lightning-quick reflexes, and deep-pattern memorization. It's challenging at times, frustrating, but damn, it makes you happy and satisfied when you win.

This is the reason why so many people, myself included, are enthralled with the television show *Ninja Warrior* (*Sasuke* in Japan). In this show, you'll see some of the most incredible athletes competing to complete the world's most challenging obstacle course. It's so difficult, that after over ten years and thousands of competitors, only a handful of people have ever completed all four stages. What makes these incredible athletes so amazing is that they all have normal day jobs too! *Ninja Warrior* champion Makoto Nagano, my personal favorite, is a fishing boat captain. The most recent *Ninja Warrior* champion, Bunpei Shiratori, is a shoe salesman! In September 2015, the show crowned its first American *Ninja Warrior* Champion: Isaac Caldiero, who works as a bus boy when he's not training. Regardless of how you spend your daytime hours to pay the bills, your alter ego can tackle missions that challenge you mentally and physically and leave you with an immense level of satisfaction.

What *Ninja Warrior* has taught me is that even those of us with challenging schedules, demanding jobs, and family commitments can make growth, challenges, and happiness a realistic goal. It simply requires an understanding of how we can become happy, and an understanding of the desire and ability to make the things that make us happy a priority in our daily lives. That could mean working on a language for 15 minutes each afternoon, taking a weekly lesson in a new musical instrument, attending a cooking class with a loved one, or finding time to work on a hobby that makes us lose track of time.

Despite what you've heard or been led to believe, you don't have to be miserable like the strong majority who are unsatisfied with their jobs. In fact, there are jobs out there that are damn fun too! Lydia Winters is a proud member of The Rebellion and is also the Director of Fun for Mojang, the company behind *Minecraft*. She attends *Minecraft* events all over the world, communicates with the community, and has a freaking blast doing so. You don't need to be unhappy, and you don't need to "suck it up" and be thankful you have a job if it leaves you completely unfulfilled and offers no room for you to grow and make progress! You simply have to elevate what you expect out of yourself, and then take daily steps to build your world around the things that make you feel alive, be it a career in video game development, customer relations, fixing cars, helping people, or anything in between. Finding your dream job or building your own business are outside the scope of this book, but I'll share my favorite resources at the end of the book in case you decide this is the path for you.

Okay, so now we have our basic framework for happiness:

* Time spent daily, hopefully in a job that challenges us, but also in our after-hours hobbies.
* An ability to show ourselves that we are making consistent progress and improvements toward a specified goal.
* Energy and attention dedicated each day to an activity that puts us in the zone.

Just as these are the things that bring us an addictive happiness in video games, they are also the things that bring us an addictive happiness in real life. Thus, these are the things we're going to prioritize and build our life around. It's time to start setting our proper goals and expectations and setting ourselves up to win. It makes our story much better, and our superhero alter egos will thank us for it.

CROSSING THE THRESHOLD— DESIGN YOUR GAME

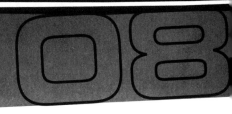

WORLD BUILDING 101: CREATE THE RULES FOR YOUR GAME OF LIFE

YOU HAVE TO LEARN THE RULES OF THE GAME. AND THEN YOU HAVE TO PLAY BETTER THAN ANYONE ELSE.

—ALBERT EINSTEIN

Ready to get your hands dirty? We have work to do! We've accepted the call to action to get started on a life structured and prioritized around the things that are important to us. We know that, just like other superheroes, we'll always have a day job and other responsibilities to return to between going on journeys and missions. But our alter egos have a responsibility to remind us that life is meant to be lived and enjoyed, too. If this is our origin story, we know there's a transformation that needs to happen.

However, we're missing a key piece of the puzzle: What is

the world like in the game we're building? What are the rules we plan on playing by that make the plot advance? If you've gotten a chance to play games like *Minecraft* or *Little Big Planet*, then you're familiar with this concept of world building: you get to place the characters, build the mountains and rivers and valleys, and then set your creations loose and role-play as your character in that world. Does it take place in Middle Earth, in which elves and orcs are battling? Is it a game in which music plays a central role—like the Ocarina in Nintendo's *The Legend of Zelda: The Ocarina of Time*? Life is a game, and we get to design the world in which we want to live. In the Hero's Journey, this is the supernatural world, or the unknown world we live in as superheroes or characters.

Here are a few familiar examples:

* Harry Potter might be an orphan who lives under the stairs, but it turns out that he's part of a much larger universe of undercover wizards, and magic is real! These rules govern how the books play out and how the story progresses.

* To those trapped in the Matrix, they are just living out a normal life. But to Neo, he is a character playing a role in the Matrix, and he gets to break rules and bend others. Oh, and he can dodge bullets and learn kung fu by downloading a program directly to his brain.

* In The Lord of the Rings, wizards help hobbits complete major tasks; orcs and goblins threaten our existence; and elves live forever unless killed in battle or die from grief or heartbreak.

How can we learn from these worlds and stories? Well, every day we have two options: we can choose to believe life is a series of random coincidences that are mostly out of our control, or we can choose to believe the world in which we live is full of secrets, that everything is epic, and that we are playing the role of a character in a massive world built around us, as characters who are on their own Hero's Journey or are helping us with ours.

Let's take it a step further. Suppose:

* You're not just walking through a city from work to the post office to mail a rent check, but you're a secret agent in a world of espionage tasked with completing a secret mission that could have dire consequences for the entire world.

* You're not just a programmer for a big corporation, but rather a superhero playing the role of a programmer, and you're playing that role to the best of your ability. You're a hacker who is finding solutions to world-changing problems during the day, and then you get to live out your alter ego at night: a dancing phenom, a musical talent, or a mixed-martial-arts master.

* You're not just exercising because you want to lose a few pounds, but because you're gathering footage for a montage of your character becoming a strong warrior who will change the fate of Middle Earth.

* You aren't reading books just to get smarter, but rather reading tomes of ancient wisdom to improve your spell-casting abilities as an all-powerful wizard.

Sure, all of the above might sound ridiculous to some, but those people are boring, and who honestly cares? People take life way too seriously, and they're not having nearly as much fun as those of us in The Rebellion who are opting out of the mundane. Here are some examples from Nerd Fitness about the Rules of The Rebellion, which govern exactly how we chose to live our lives. Obviously, with it being a fitness site these are going to have a bit of a health-slant to them, but they give us the rules that govern our decisions every day to maximize fun, health, growth, and adventure (you can see the full rules and descriptions at NerdFitness.com/Rules):

1. **We don't care where you came from, only where you're going.** We don't care where you came from or how you got here, as we all have different backgrounds, genetics, social

status, and commitments. Like creating a random character in a role-playing game, we were all "dealt a hand" that we had absolutely no control over—it's now up to us to play that hand to the best of our ability. This is a kick-ass group of people pushing each other to level up our lives. We figure out what went wrong, and then we work together to find a way to fix it. The past is just that: the past. Today can be the first day of the rest of your life if you truly believe that.

2. **When you join, you're in for life.** We aren't looking for quick fixes or for people who aren't interested in making permanent lasting changes. The Rebellion is full of people who are interested in prioritizing adventure, happiness, and improvement. If your friends won't join you on your mission, then you'll have to lead by example until they decide to follow. It's a heavy burden to bear, but one that will absolutely make your life more fulfilling.

3. **We train as naturally as possible.** When we train for adventure, we do so by preparing our bodies with real-world movements! We don't use machines; we focus on movements that recruit multiple muscle groups and efficiently set us up to be antifragile (don't worry, I cover this in detail later in the book).

4. **We take care of our nutrition.** How we fuel our bodies is 80 percent of the battle and will determine how successful we will be on the battlefield of life. I'm not talking about switching to all salads and water, but small, calculated changes to what you eat over a long period of time. We understand that although the total number of calories we eat certainly impacts our health, WHAT those calories are made of is just as important, if not more so.

5. **We train with conviction and intelligence.** When exercising, we have a plan for what we're going to do, and we know how hard we need to push ourselves to be better than the day before. When setting life goals, we have a plan for what we're going to do, and what needs to be accomplished in order for

us to make progress. Then, we do it. We plan out what kind of superhero we want to be, pick our own super power, and work every day toward becoming that hero. Those who are willing to dedicate themselves to the cause will get results. Settling is not an option.

6. **We exercise because it's fun.** Find something that makes you happy, gets your heart pumping, and will keep you in shape. There is something out there for everybody, so keep searching and keep pushing until you find something that drives you to succeed. Yoga, karate, cycling, Belegarth, whatever it is—find it and do it. This is a crucial part of an adventurous life!

7. **We never leave our wingmen.** We're all in this together, and we're here to support each other. Although we have friendly competitions, it's all in good fun to keep us accountable.

    If you are training or leveling up your life with friends in real life or online, pick them up when they're down, motivate them when they're tired, push them when they need encouragement, and yell when they need tough love. They'll do the same for you one day, and we'll all be better off because of it. Never leave your wingman.

8. **We question everything.** The Rebellion exists to open our minds to a world in which the impossible is possible. We want to show you a world you didn't even know existed, like the Matrix. We question conventional wisdom and social norms and "because that's how it's always been done," and we find our own path. It's then up to us to take what we've learned, question it, and find a way to apply it to our lives.

9. **We take care of business.** If you're a gamer, keep gaming. If you're a family man, you better show up at your kid's soccer game instead of staying late at work. We all have things we love in life, things that are important to us, that make us who we are. As long as these things aren't detrimental to our health, then I encourage you to keep doing them. We also have obligations to

our families, employers, and friends—we do what we say and we say what we do.

10. **We take pride in ourselves.** Too many people blame their unfortunate situation on the government, the weather, their genetics, global warming, the economy, their parents, etc. Not us. We don't expect anything to be handed to us; we are not owed anything by anybody. In fact, it's our responsibility as humans to live the best life possible. We want to be better husbands, wives, fathers, mothers, sons, daughters, people. We want to be stronger, faster, and healthier—we know it's going to take a lot of hard work and determination to get there. *We welcome the challenge.*

Whenever we're not sure what needs to happen next, or if we have a difficult decision to make, we can refer back to these rules, which tell us how our game works. They give our world a set of constructs to live by, and they give us a chance to simplify every step we take every day, down to these essentials. And we have fun with it!

After all, we all need more fun in our lives, and everything gets more fun and epic when we look at it as though the world in which we live has been built from the ground up with ourselves as the main character. You are the character this story is built around, and everybody is pulling for you to succeed. What's that? You want to be the Han to Luke Skywalker? Hermione to Harry Potter? That's fine too—it's your world and your life! You get to set the rules, and the guidelines that you chose to live by.

So start thinking about your game world from a much higher level. Build your world and superhero's story around the things you've chosen to prioritize. I personally wanted to live a life of adventure and music, so I've decided I'm living in a world in which anything is possible, where adventure is hiding around every corner, and music plays a central role in my growth and happiness, too.

Remember, the choice is yours as to how to attack the things that need to get done every day, and the world in which you live is shaped by how you view it. It's either a daring adventure or nothing at all. We members of The Rebellion choose to look at life like it's a big, freaking adventure and everything is epic. Now that we've established we're living in a world in which anything is possible, it's time to look at the Hero's Journey of our character and, specifically, what type of avatar we're building.

To the character-creation screen!

REBEL HERO

★ ★ ★ ★ ★ ★

NAME: *Shannon Andrews*   AGE: *30*

HOMETOWN: *Minneapolis, MN*

I'm a physician in training: crazy schedules, fragmented sleep, and a shaky support system. Life continually spiraled out of control leading to shortcuts with my health. The Rebellion became a safe haven amidst the chaos, especially once I found my guild home—the assassins. Slowly, a group of parkour moms, amateur circus artists, hedonistic home chefs, and new recruits became my Fellowship.

Their camaraderie helped me experiment with small sustainable changes out of which grew three new passions—mindfulness, cooking, and hiking. Although the assassins are my home, I took many vacations with the druids to practice mindfulness. They were patient and steady as I practiced this new discipline. This fundamentally changed my mindset while leveling up.

Mindfulness allows me to step away from perfectionism long enough to choose the path of self-compassion instead. Meditation is a daily habit for me now.

For decades, I rebelled against traditional gender roles. The Rebellion was full of people preparing meals, and I soon found that I love to cook, preferably from scratch. Eating my own food was cheaper and better than eating in restaurants (not to mention eating in pajamas)! Each challenge I discovered new secrets like slow cookers, batch cooking, and freedom

SPOTLIGHT

DAY JOB: *Physician*

ALTER EGO: *Anny Shay*   **CLASS:** *Assassin*

from counting calories. Slowly these secrets became habits, and I'm enjoying food instead of fighting against it.

I've always loved to hike, but the discipline that I was learning in The Rebellion got me thinking that I could tackle something more epic. After all, if Sam and Frodo could get to Mount Doom, what mountain couldn't I tackle? My roommate and I set our sights on completing the Presidential Traverse. I used multiple challenges to prepare while Rebels were cheering each step. In September of 2014, we trekked the Presidential Traverse in three days. It was the first time either of us had backpacked, and we learned A TON. That is one of the biggest victories of my life, since it proved to me how strong and capable I am. Currently, I'm playing with craving-control habits, locomotive movement, and swing dance. After all, winter is coming and a Rebel needs to keep moving to stay warm!

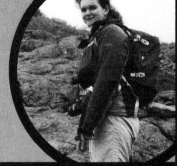

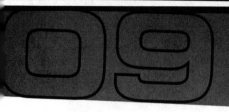

CHARACTER SELECT: DETERMINE YOUR "LEVEL 50" ACHIEVEMENT STATUS

READY PLAYER ONE.   *—EVERY VIDEO GAME, EVER*

I want you to imagine life for the superhero/adventure character you've created when he/she is operating at the highest level of bad-assery.

Think of role-playing games where we spend the whole game leveling up our character to the max level so we can slay dragons and complete world-changing missions. Sure, we might start out with just a cloth tunic and rusted dagger, but we know if we stick with it long enough, we can eventually reach the max level and become a strong warrior, master ranger, awe-inspiring wizard, or stealthy assassin. And life is pretty great at Level 50: you get to enter special zones, wear special armor, and the level comes with a certain amount of prestige. Oh, and you can pretty much vanquish any bad guy you want.

Why should life be any different? We've built a world in which we want our character to live; we have determined the rules that govern the game; and now we need to determine just what type of character our hero will be! In games, there are a million different combinations that can result in a max-level character, and life is no different. You can be a battle mage who is equally strong and wise, casting lightning bolts with one hand and swinging a flaming sword with the other. Another character might play the same game completely differently, though, and create a drastically different type of character at Level 50.

It's time to start physically constructing your personal avatar—your alter ego. I want you to determine what type of character you hope to be when you reach your personal Level 50. Depending on your current situation, your "max level" might be simple or extraordinary. You might be focused on getting healthy, or traveling, or increasing your wisdom and intelligence, or simply giving back. In order to get this process started, I want to share with you a few archetypes you can use to help determine what type of character you want to become.

Ultimately, I want you think of how you would answer the question that King Leonidas of Sparta asked his faithful 300 warriors: "What is your profession?" And I don't mean, "What do you do for a living?"; but rather, "How does your character view this world of adventure?" Even if you are a couch potato who has never gone on an adventure, I want you to pick what kind of character you WANT to be and then we'll work on getting you there. After all, it's tough to adventure if we're not built for it!

I always start by encouraging heroes to pick the type of activity he or she plans on pursuing when it comes to adventure. We're designed to move, and thus a healthy body is a happy body: We need to find a way to introduce physical adventure into our lives if we're going to live up to our full potential. We can't take on the world if we can't first get off the couch or if we get winded after climbing a flight of stairs!

Below is how the class system is built in The Rebellion at Nerd Fitness. This gives us a great starting point around which to start prioritizing our adventures, quests, and missions. You can create your character and pick your class at LevelUpYourLife.com.

CLASS ARCHETYPES

WARRIOR: You love the idea of getting stronger and more powerful. Every day is an opportunity to move heavy things or test yourself against others in competition and prove your might.

* **Fictional example:** Thor of Asgard (*The Avengers*), Maximus Decimus Meridius (*Gladiator*), Brienne of Tarth (*Game of Thrones*)

* **Real-world example:** Hafthór Júlíus "Thor" Björnsson, who plays "The Mountain" on *Game of Thrones*

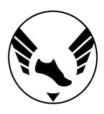

SCOUT: Built for distance and efficiency rather than strength and power, you can outlast any animal on the planet. Your muscles are designed with endurance in mind, and you can cover great distances whenever necessary.

* **Fictional example:** Legolas of the Woodland Realm (The Lord of the Rings)

* **Real-world example:** Rita Jeptoo, Boston Marathon record holder; Jan Frodeno, 2008 Olympic gold medalist and 2015 Ironman champion

RANGER: A jack-of-all-trades, Rangers are well-equipped for any situation. You're good at strength training and pretty good at covering distances when required, but neither is a specialty.

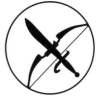

* **Fictional example:** Jon Snow (*Game of Thrones*), Katniss Everdeen (The Hunger Games)
* **Real-world example:** Rich Froning Jr., four-time winner of the CrossFit Games

ASSASSIN: Every building can be climbed, every gap can be jumped, every obstacle can be conquered. Assassins spend most of their time training with functional body-weight exercises, as that's usually the only thing they need to lift. Gymnasts and parkour enthusiasts would fit into this category.

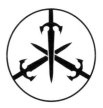

* **Fictional example:** Ezio Auditore (*Assassin's Creed 2*)
* **Real-world example:** Kacy Catanzaro of *American Ninja Warrior* fame; Damien Walters, professional stuntman, gymnastics coach, and free-running professional

MONK: Monks can kick your ass with their fists and feet, and they can do it before you even know what's happened. Incredibly agile, lightning fast, and loaded with power, Monks specialize in martial arts to stay in shape and destroy the opposition.

* **Fictional example:** Neo (*The Matrix*); Beatrix Kiddo aka Black Mamba (*Kill Bill*)
* **Real-world example:** UFC fighters Georges St-Pierre and Ronda Rousey

DRUID: Druids spend a majority of their time training in the arts of yoga, tai chi, and other movement-based disciplines. Each movement has a purpose, and that purpose is to further improve the dexterity, agility, and strength of the druid.

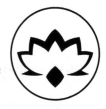

* **Fictional example:** Lady Galadriel (The Lord of the Rings)
* **Real-world example:** Josh Waitzkin, Tai Chi Push Hands US champion and chess prodigy

ADVENTURER: Adventurers are brave souls who fear nothing and are always curious about what's over the next hill or across the ocean. They are often found working diligently with their allies to help ensure that every adventure leads down the correct path, exploring and learning for the sake of others.

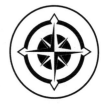

* **Fictional example:** Indiana Jones, Lara Croft (*Tomb Raider*)
* **Real-world example:** Les Stroud (*Survivorman*); Lewis and Clark, explorers

Now, these are simply some fun archetypes to get the ball rolling. The great news is, there's no wrong way to play Life when it's an adventure, and the type of character you get to play is totally up to you. Despite what the movie *WarGames* will tell you, the only wrong way to play is to not play at all. So I want you to take a few minutes and think of your favorite way of being active. Even if you're 500 pounds and couch-bound, think about the type of character you'd like to be, or the types of activities you hope to one day complete.

Don't fit perfectly into one of the categories above? Great. Me neither! I'm more like an assassin-adventurer-bard hybrid, which I've determined is a "Troubadour." If you want to be a berserker or a battle mage, that's totally up to you. What's important is that you start to apply specific traits to the type of character you plan on building, because it helps paint a more complete picture as we move forward.

Along with our physical attributes, feel free to identify other attributes you want to associate with your character when he or she is a badass:

* Constitution
* Courage
* Intelligence
* Wisdom
* Charisma
* Humor
* Generosity

You're limited only by your imagination and the qualities you have deemed important in your life. I now want you to write out what life is like for you at your max level of 50, and be specific! It doesn't matter if you're not 100 percent sure of every tiny detail, but being specific gives us a starting point that we're then going to work on fine-tuning over the next few chapters.

Back in 2011, when I first started to build my life around the idea that it was a game, this is what I decided my Level 50 looked like:

FROM A FITNESS PERSPECTIVE, I'M IN THE BEST SHAPE OF MY LIFE—HANDSTAND PUSH-UPS, PISTOL SQUATS, PULL-UPS, AND A 405-POUND DEADLIFT. I'M ALSO FLEXIBLE AS HELL, WELL TRAINED IN KUNG FU, A GREAT BREAK-DANCER, AND A DAMN GOOD COOK. I LIVE IN A NICE HOUSE ON THE COAST. I WAKE UP WITHOUT AN ALARM CLOCK AND GRAB MY SURFBOARD FOR A MORNING SESSION.

I SPEND THE MIDDLE OF MY DAY WORKING ON NERD FITNESS AND THE REBELLION (WHILE ALSO BOOKING A BUSI-NESS TRIP TO . . . HAWAII? JAPAN? AND A FREE VACATION TO

TAHITI USING AIRLINE MILES), AND THEN SNEAK OUT TO PLAY SOME GOLF IN THE AFTERNOON AT A LOCAL COURSE. I COME HOME, CRANK OUT A QUICK STRENGTH-TRAINING WORKOUT OR MARTIAL-ARTS SESSION, COOK A HEALTHY DINNER FOR MY WIFE AND MYSELF, AND THEN RELAX BY INVITING SOME FRIENDS OVER FOR DRINKS, MUSIC, CARDS AGAINST HUMANITY, AND HANGING OUT.

That was the life I wanted to live at Level 50 a few years back. Here I am today, and some of my goals have certainly shifted a bit. I'm sure a few years from now they'll shift again. And that's fine! I'm not at Level 50 yet, but I'm much closer now to the life I hope to live than I was back then! Every time I go out on a quest or a mission, I return with a fun story I'll never forget, a transformed perspective about what's important to me, and the desire to make some adjustments and get closer to those goals. These two paragraphs gave me a starting point and something to work toward as I was developing myself as a hero. Most important, it gave me permission to take action because I had a direction in which to go.

Take another few minutes right now and write out two paragraphs on what life is like for you at Level 50. What are your main attributes? How is your time spent? Do you wake up and train in your favorite martial art before taking your kids to school? Do you prepare a world-class meal for your family and neighbors every night? Do you work at your own restaurant and then go surfing? Do you code with friends on a game you're building and then come home to practice with your band in the garage?

The more specific you can be, the better. Even if your life at Level 50 seems drastically distant at this point, I still want you to participate.

Here is my character at Level 50 goals right now, in 2015:

NAME: STEVE KAMB
ALTER EGO: REBEL ONE
LIFE AT LEVEL 50: LIVING IN A HOUSE ON A COASTLINE, UP EARLY WITH THE SUNRISE TO WRITE ARTICLES OR WORK

ON MY NEXT BOOK. LATE MORNING IS SPENT AT THE GYM TRAINING WITH POWERLIFTING, GYMNASTICS, AND CAPOEIRA EXERCISES. MY AFTERNOONS ARE SPENT PLAYING GOLF OR MUSIC UNTIL MY KIDS COME HOME FROM SCHOOL. MY EVENINGS ARE SPENT WITH FAMILY AND/OR FRIENDS, EAT-ING A HOME-COOKED DINNER OUTSIDE AROUND A FIRE, LIVE MUSIC BEING PLAYED, AND FUN BEING HAD BY ALL. WHEN I'M NOT AT HOME LIVING MY LIFE, I'M TRAVELING ON AN IMPORTANT MISSION OR ADVENTURE THAT CHALLENGES ME PHYSICALLY AND MENTALLY.

Go now to LevelUpYourLife.com, where you can create your own character, and fill out your personal profile and attributes. In the next chapter we'll get into the actual quest/mission portion of the game you're building, which you can do online, too!

If you're struggling to come up with the type of character you want to be, feel free to look at real-life people who are where you want to be. When you are playing a game like *World of Warcraft* and you are at Level 1, looking at somebody who is Level 50 inspires you to get started; one look at his inventory and you're inspired to play more. You know it took this guy months or years of questing, grinding, and dungeon crawling, but if he can get to Level 50 and get all that stuff, so can you some day. Having that model to look at gives us a chance to say, "Okay, he did it! And I'm not going to get any closer standing here. I might as well get started."

You already know my imaginary inspirational characters, but my real-life inspiration is Richard Branson, founder of Virgin. In my mind, Richard has prioritized the Game of Life, and built an incredibly successful business around his idea of fun, adventure, and disrupting the status quo. He also enjoys every day, making sure to give back where he can, reminding himself that it's a great day to be alive and adventure is out there for those who seek it. Oh, and he owns his own island!

Earlier in this book you read the story of Megan, the world-traveling school teacher, and maybe thought to yourself, "Hey, that does sound like fun, I'd like to do that, too!" Or maybe as you read the stories of the Rebels throughout this book, you're realizing there are people who have similar situations to you, and they are doing things you've always wanted to do.

Who are some people who are living the Level 50 life that you'd like to live similarly to? Is there a guy your age who picked up a new instrument or learned a new language? Do you know somebody who has traveled to a country you've always wanted to visit? How about that woman who has had a dramatic weight-loss success, while juggling a hectic life as a single mom?

Some might look at these Level 50 characters and say things like, "Must be nice." Members of The Rebellion look at them and say, "If they can do it, so can I!" As to how we're going to get from Level 1 to Level 50, that's why you're reading this strategy guide! For each of the attributes of the life you want to live, we can identify specific missions and types of quests that will get us to Level 50. The end result is an adventurous and rewarding life.

QUEST SELECT: CHOOSE YOUR OWN ADVENTURE

THE CHOICE IS YOURS, AND YOURS ALONE.

—*OLMEC,* LEGENDS OF THE HIDDEN TEMPLE

In *The Legend of Zelda,* your main quest as Link is to collect the Triforce, defeat Ganon, rescue Princess Zelda, and save Hyrule. However, along the way there are dozens of side quests that can occupy your time. Whether it's fishing in Lake Hylia, collecting heart pieces, winning at the archery mini-game, rescuing chickens, or solving puzzles, there are always things to be done, and fun tasks to complete.

The same is true for *World of Warcraft,* a game composed of thousands of quests. You might be working on a big master quest, but there are always side quests that help you earn experience points, discover new locations, find new items, craft new armor, level up certain attributes, and so on. These quests can be a fun distraction, can improve your character in different ways, or even make the master quest easier by unlocking shortcuts.

In a similar vein, we're going to get started with building our very own list of quests. These are the missions we'll need to accomplish in order for us to level up our primary attributes and actually level up our lives! Just as we needed to be specific in describing the Level 50 character we plan to create, we also need to get specific as to how we plan to get there. When our quests are concrete (specific things that we can check off our lists and say, "Quest complete") we're going to have a much clearer path to success. Let me give you a few basic examples:

* If strength is one of the key attributes that you wish to level up, then "Get strong" is too vague a goal. Better to set a specific fitness goal like "execute a 300-pound deadlift" or "hold a handstand for 60 seconds"; "do 10 pull-ups" or "compete in a powerlifting competition."

* If your goal is to level up your wisdom or constitution attribute, "Learn French" is simply too broad. Instead, something like, "Have a conversation completely in French with a native speaker while in Paris" is more effective. When you arrive in Paris and only speak French to your cab driver to get safely from the airport to your hotel, you can then check off this quest. DING!

* "Travel more" won't do much to level up your courage attribute! Now, "Visit the Bioluminescent Bay off the coast of Vieques in Puerto Rico by April 2020" is far more specific, and gives you a chance to start preparing to make that goal into a reality.

You might notice that those three example quests operate completely independent of one another. And why not? Who says you can't travel to amazing places while learning a new language and getting better at pull-ups in your game? I've chosen to break my own Game of Life into different categories for ease of sorting, which I'll share with you shortly. Whenever I struggle to come up with new ideas, I look to my favorite games, books, and movies for inspiration and have a blast trying to create real-life scenarios that pay homage to those adventures. It often results in something ridiculous, like flying a stunt plane, living like James Bond, taking swing-dance classes, or being an extra on a TV show.

By having a list that's varied, diverse, and challenging, you'll be leveling up your life in many different ways. Essentially, you're turning yourself into a modern-day Renaissance Man/Woman. Let's take a look at some sample categories and examples. It doesn't matter if these quests are massive and seem light years away from completion. We need to start somewhere, and we're going to start by creating our quest system. There are 10 different categories below, and I want you to put five quests in each category. Visit LevelUpYourLife.com to create your own list, assign point values, and start to level up your life.

1. PHYSICAL QUESTS

These are quests that challenge you physically and require you to level up your health and wellness in some way. I've been running a health and fitness site for over six years, so this is probably one of my most important categories. I personally believe a strong body is a healthy body, and strength on the outside can help create inner strength and confidence, so my goals revolve around strength training. On top of that, I know how important it is to take care of your body if you are interested in accomplishing lots of goals in your life.

EXAMPLES:

* Run the Boston Marathon.
* Hold a handstand for 60 seconds.
* Deadlift 405 lbs (183 kg).
* Earn a black belt in tai kwon do.
* Climb Mount Kilimanjaro.

2. MENTAL QUESTS

As Ben Stiller's character says in the film *Dodgeball,* "I like to break a mental sweat, too"; or, as Morpheus says in *The Matrix,* "the body cannot exist without the mind." These are quests that challenge your brain, make you smarter, or give you a chance to operate on a higher intellectual level.

EXAMPLES:

* Have a 30 minute conversation in Spanish with a native speaker.
* Memorize the order of an entire deck of cards.
* Successfully develop and launch an iPhone application.
* Take six months of weekly lessons on the bagpipes.
* Earn a college degree.

3. FUN QUESTS

When was the last time you set aside time to do things, purely for the fun of it? Life is damn short, and we need to spend time every day doing things that make us happy. These are things we've always said we wanted to do, but never had time for.

EXAMPLES:

* Sign up for swing-dance classes with a partner.
* Paint a picture a week for a month.
* Attend Comic-Con in full costume—one you made yourself.
* Take a cooking class at the local culinary school.
* Skip work one day and have your kids play hooky and build a pillow fort.

4. WORK QUESTS

We've spent quite a bit of time talking about things that make us happy or make us feel alive, but we also need to make sure we pay the bills, too, or our alter ego will never get a chance to level up. Sure, it would be nice to say "just follow your passion and build a business," but things are often more complicated than that. Maybe you have specific goals when it comes to your business, your job, or your career. Ultimately, the goal is to reverse-engineer your life and your work AROUND the adventure, instead of trying to cram adventure into a few days of vacation every year.

EXAMPLES:

* Publish a fantasy novel.
* Exhibit a work of art in a gallery.
* Have five consulting clients.
* Make a six-figure salary.
* Get a job as a [insert awesome job here].

5. ADVENTURE QUESTS

I had never been outside North America before I started my Epic Quest of Awesome, but I had always LOVED movies like those in the Indiana Jones series. I would watch that red line fly around the globe and imagine myself visiting far off locations, exploring ancient ruins, and more. So, when I began traveling, that's where I started with my list: not just "to travel," but rather to become a real-life Indiana Jones or Nathan Drake from the Uncharted series. These can be locations in your own town or state, or in the far corners of the globe. If the Goonies can find adventure in their backyard, so can you.

EXAMPLES:

* Visit the ruins of Machu Picchu in Peru.
* Hike 10 mapped trails in your hometown.
* Explore Petra, Jordan (*Indiana Jones and the Last Crusade!*).
* Stay in a castle in Scotland.
* Drive across country with your college friends.

6. COURAGE QUESTS

I'm pretty much a risk-averse nerd, and lots of stuff scares the crap out of me, which is exactly why I make myself do it! I said yes to every public speaking offer that came my way before I could talk myself out of it, because I'm terrified of public speaking! Maybe you have fear or anxiety about talking to people, performing in public, or maybe even asking for somebody's phone number. It's up to you to determine what kinds of quests scare the crap out of you.

EXAMPLES:

* Give a talk to 50 or more people.
* Ask for one person's phone number every day this week.
* Do five minutes of stand-up comedy.
* Strike up a conversation with a complete stranger.
* Sing a five-song set on a street corner.

7. FREEDOM QUESTS

These are quests that would allow you to spend more time with friends and family on things you enjoy doing. It might be finding a way to be mobile with your current job, or negotiating more time off, or quitting and actually doing what you want to do with your life. Ultimately, if we are going to live our lives like an adventure game, we need to build our lives around that game. Because my game involved me becoming Indiana Jones, I needed to create a mobile business focused on helping people.

EXAMPLES:

* Negotiate a day to work from home each week.
* Get out of debt.
* Get four weeks of vacation instead of three.
* Create an online business that generates $1,000 a month on the side.
* Work remotely and travel with your partner for six weeks.

8. MASTER QUESTS

Every RPG seems to have those MASSIVE master quests that come at the end of the game. These quests require you to scour the planet or defeat the highest-level dragon to create the ultimate piece of armor, or mine some ultra-rare mineral from the bottom of a cave to craft the ultimate flaming sword. In real life, we can have master quests, too. These are quests that might be ridiculous or seem like a long ways off, but also happen to be a lot of fun or include a significant life event. Remember to be specific with these, too.

EXAMPLES:

* Get married.
* Buy a house that overlooks the ocean.
* Experience zero gravity.
* Fly around the world in a hot air balloon.
* Visit every country on the planet.

9. GRATITUDE QUESTS

One of my favorite parts of playing massively multiplayer games is helping out other characters who are at lower levels than I am. At Nerd Fitness I love doing what I can with our community to raise money or awareness for great causes, too. I think giving back to our fellow gamers or to those who can't help themselves is incredibly important, and many people have built their entire Game of Life around this concept! You can think as grand or small as you'd like for this and have fun with it!

EXAMPLES:

* Spend a week volunteering at an orphanage.
* Raise $10,000 for a charity that's important to you.
* Cook a meal for a needy family on Thanksgiving.
* Raise enough money to build a well in Africa through Charity: Water.
* Pay $100 for a glass of lemonade from the neighbor's kid.

CONTINUED ON PAGE 104

REBEL HERO

★ ★ ★ ★ ★ ★

NAME: *Thomas Sorensen*   AGE: 57

HOMETOWN: *Carson City, NV*

I owe a lot of my success, particularly in the martial arts, to Steve's concept of "gamifying your life." As a single parent, I often found myself overwhelmed with tasks and issues requiring my attention. Then, about a year ago, I stumbled across an apparently popular story called *Lone Wolf and Cub*, a story about a single father trying to raise his son in the face of many difficulties.

It occurred to me that there were a lot of similarities between myself and Ogami Itto. We were both single fathers determined to redeem our honor. We were both martial artists with a deep respect for the warrior code, and yet we were both willing to break that code to ensure the survival of our sons and the completion of our quests.

I combined my love of video games with my love of the Lone Wolf and Cub series. It occurred to me one day that I could arrange every single task and issue that I had in my life into a sort of daily quest log, and adjust my priorities accordingly, simplifying life and allowing me to become more efficient.

It was also around this time that I rekindled my old love for the martial arts. I dove in with a passion, seeking out every source of knowledge that I could find. I spent time researching everything and putting what I found to the test until I found what worked. The results were astounding—not only did

SPOTLIGHT

DAY JOB: Construction Manager

ALTER EGO: Aegis   **CLASS:** Samurai

I remember what I had been taught, but I now had the ability to see the practical applications of techniques as well as understand the philosophical views of the old masters. I learned more having to figure things out for myself than I ever could have learned in a *dojo*.

I have begun teaching my son Karate-do. At the first lesson I found that not only was I was able to teach Karate-do naturally, but I also had an unexpected depth and breadth of knowledge—and I owed it all to the thousands of hours spent training with my *sensei* all those years ago. Teaching my son is a continuously rewarding experience, and I find that I learn much about myself and my own practice from teaching him.

In addition to excelling in Karate-do, I took up the practice of freestyle *kenjutsu*, as well as qi gong, yoga, and Yang-style tai chi. I practice the sword often, and I find that many of the skills that are useful in Karate-do translate nicely into *kenjutsu*. My son and I take each day as it comes, much like Ogami Itto and his son Daigoro, and we keep going one step at a time.

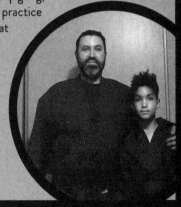

10. LEGACY QUESTS

This is a bit of an unusual category, but we all want to leave the world a better place, right? And we might want to be known for something that made a lasting impact on those around us. It can be what we're known for on a grand scale, or simply how we hope those who know us best will remember us.

EXAMPLES:

* Write a *New York Times* bestselling book.
* Record an album that gets at least 1,000 downloads on iTunes.
* Set a world record recognized by Guinness.
* Earn enough so that your child can attend four years of college without incurring massive student loans.
* Pay for a trip for all of your grandchildren to visit Disney World with you.

Feel free to take out a piece of notebook paper, open up a Word document, or go to LevelUpYourLife.com, and spend a few minutes dreaming up a preliminary list of quests you'd like to complete. If any of the previous categories don't align with the goals or attributes you're aiming for, feel free to make up your own category. Love music? Put a greater focus on music quests. Or maybe you want to learn a new martial art every few years: create a quest based around that! You're only limited by your imagination!

Don't worry if you decide down the road that you need to change quests, or your life situation changes drastically and you need to switch the game you're playing. What's important is to identify our quests and know what type of character we want to build so that we can actually start to take steps toward leveling up a reality.

STEVE'S EPIC QUEST: LEARN FROM MY EXAMPLE

LIFE IS EITHER A DARING ADVENTURE OR NOTHING AT ALL.
—HELEN KELLER

The *Epic Quest of Awesome* is the name I've chosen to give to my Game of Life. I started my quest list back in 2010 because I needed some inspiration to get off my butt and start thinking on a much grander scale. Although my quest initially revolved mostly around travel, it has evolved over time as new hobbies have developed and new events have taken place. Less emphasis has been placed on being nomadic and more has been placed on personal development. Originally, I organized my quests by travel zones. Each continent became a "zone" like you'd find in adventure games. There was the desert zone (Africa), the jungle zone (South America), the water zone (South Pacific/Australia), the newbie zone (North America).

As I started to spend more and more time on my quest, though, I began to add to it more and more categories that fit in with what I hoped to accomplish, and I jettisoned others that didn't fit quite so well. The quest, like you, is a work in progress, and the adaptability of the quest is part of what makes it so awesome. If your goals or priorities change, you can still build your game and your list of quests around the things that are important to you. You shouldn't ever be afraid to evolve the game, drop quests, or change them up if your life changes.

Allow me to share with you a sampling of the Hero Quests I created for myself as part of my overarching Epic Quest of Awesome. You'll notice I organized these into various quest types to focus on certain attributes I want to improve or experiences I want to have.

Along with the quest itself, there are also rewards associated with the completion of certain boss battles. As with any game, I make sure to reward myself with items that reward me back. For example, if I complete enough music quests I might unlock a new guitar—which would then inspire and encourage me to spend more time playing and improving!

Below are the different categories of quests I've built my life around, including a few sample quests in each. You can see the full list and my progress at LevelUpYourLife.com. The fun part is that this is uniquely mine. You might look at some items on this list and think "I could never do that!" while others might make you say, "That's easy, Steve, how have you not done that yet?" We're all at different levels, and everything we work on is a challenge.

1. PHYSICAL QUESTS

A lot of my life revolves around being physically active, as it's what I spend my days working on over at NerdFitness.com. But just as my interests are varied so, too, are my physical goals and missions. I like to level up my strength in two ways: power lifting and bodyweight manipulation. This is how I train daily, so it's how my goals are organized.

* Hold a free handstand for 60 seconds.
* Deadlift 405 lbs (183 kg).
* Complete 10 pull-ups with 50 extra pounds (22 kg).
* Complete 10 one-arm pushups with each arm.
* Participate in a Brazilian capoeira roda—think of it like a breakdance fight/dance in a circle.

2. JASON BOURNE QUESTS

I am a massive fan of Jason Bourne as a character. I just love the concept of being able to go anywhere, do anything, and disappear at the drop of a hat. He is truly the most antifragile character out there—he can get himself into and out of any situation. Multiple languages, foreign bank accounts, parkour skill, and more. How cool is that!?

* Have a conversation in a foreign country with a native speaker (learn a second language; done!)
* Build a bug-out bag, and spend a weekend living out of it exclusively.
* Learn how to pick the lock on a pair of handcuffs.
* Obtain a second passport.
* Spend six months training in Krav Maga (martial art).

3. FUN QUESTS

Life is too damn short, so we need to make sure we are having fun on a daily basis. Otherwise, what's the point? I tend to get caught up too much in my work or training and need to remind myself sometimes to let loose, drink a few beers, and go do something really fun.

* Attend La Tomatina in Spain—the tomato-throwing festival.
* Attend Oktoberfest in Munich, Germany (done!).
* Visit the Lagavulin distillery in Scotland.
* Attend Comic-Con in full costume.
* Play Pebble Beach Golf Links with dad and brother.

4. BUSINESS QUESTS

Although I studied economics in college, my favorite courses were entrepreneurship-focused. I love the idea of being 100 percent in control of my destiny and building a business I can be proud of. I've been building Nerd Fitness for years and years, and I'm excited to continue to grow it, provide quality jobs for people who can work from anywhere, and really help people live better lives.

* Make a full-time living through Nerd Fitness (done!).
* Publish a book that becomes a *New York Times* bestseller.
* Have 500,000 subscribers to Nerd Fitness.
* Take my team at NF on a whitewater rafting trip.
* Turn Nerd Fitness into a company worth $100 million.

5. ADVENTURE QUESTS

My life has become an adventure game, so I've identified specific moments from my favorite movies and games I'd want to re-create in real life. Here are some of my quests that will take me all over the globe.

* Visit the ruins of Machu Picchu in Peru (done!).
* Find Nemo on the Great Barrier Reef (done!).
* Climb Mount Kilimanjaro in Tanzania.
* Carve my own surfboard and then ride it in Hawaii.
* Visit Antarctica.

6. COURAGE QUESTS

I'm pretty much a risk-averse nerd, which means lots of things scare me or give me anxiety. Eating foreign foods, speaking in public, performing in public, and lots of fearful activities are a good reminder that "Hey, you're alive, and it didn't kill you!"

* Bungee jump at Kawarau Bridge in New Zealand (done!).
* Perform on stage in front of more than 1,000 (done!).
* Speak at a conference with more than 2,000 people in the audience.
* Be a guest on a late night talk show.
* Dive with sharks in South Africa.

7. ROCK STAR QUESTS

I took piano lessons when I was a little kid, but never really started to enjoy playing music until I was in high school. Once I moved to Nashville (the music capital of the world) for college, I was hooked. There was just one problem—I wasn't very good! I've since put in daily effort to improve my skills at playing various instruments and singing.

* Sit at a piano in a bar, start playing "Piano Man," and by the end of the song have the whole bar singing along.
* Play violin for at least 30 minutes at a pub in Ireland.
* Play a five-song set list with my guitar on a street corner (done!).
* Write, record, and publish an original song.
* Own a baby grand piano.

8. MASTER QUESTS

There are always quests in games that carry more significance than the other quests: they might have way more steps or require hours of commitment, but the reward can be monumental. These are the quests on my list that seem absolutely ridiculous to me and would signify my Game of Life is getting crazy, which is why they are on here!

* Buy a tropical island.
* Go into outer space.
* Spend an afternoon with Sir Richard Branson.
* Get invited to the White House and meet the president.
* Be a featured extra in a Marvel movie.

9. MENTAL/SPIRITUAL QUESTS

My mind never stops working. I'm thinking about Nerd Fitness and ideas for the business nearly every waking minute of every day, and it often keeps me from getting to sleep at night! I know mental health is just as important as regular health, and it has recently become a much bigger focus for me as the stakes have gotten bigger.

* Meditate for 5 minutes every morning for 30 days straight.
* Spend a week at a meditation retreat in Southeast Asia.
* Visit a deprivation tank and float.
* Attend two yoga classes per week for a month.
* Spend a week hiking without technology.

10. GRATITUDE QUESTS

A big part of what I do with Nerd Fitness is help people help themselves to get healthy and happy. However, there are plenty of people (and animals) who can't help themselves, and I think an important part of how we spend our time can be used to help others live better lives, too.

* Volunteer weekly at a local children's hospital for at least six months (done!).
* Help build a house through Habitat for Humanity (done!)
* Raise and contribute $10 million for a charity that's important to the Nerd Fitness Community.
* Spend a week at an orphanage in a foreign country.
* Leave a $100 tip at a random late-night diner with a waiter or waitress who could really use the money.

At this point, hopefully, your brain is exploding with ideas for what you can put on your list and how you plan on creating your game. As your mentor, I hope I've shown some of the paths available to you and some of the quests and missions you can create. Now head on over to LevelUpYourLife.com and create your character, see other characters, publish your list, and get ideas from others. Your list is simply a way to get started, and start you must. Maybe you want to visit all 50 states, or learn a dance from every continent, or set a world record in handstand push-ups, or go to Mars!

There are no wrong answers, nothing too ridiculous, and nothing too far away. What's important now is to think about your favorite games, books, and movies—draw some inspiration and have some fun putting together your list. You can always add more to it. You can change quests. You can stop quests that no longer seem fun for you. As your life changes, so, too, can your quest lists.

But get going, my dear Rebel friend! For once you've created your list, we can finally get started with crossing items off our list, leveling up, and living out the adventure we've been dreaming up in the extraordinary world of our journey! Otherwise, your quest list will be nothing more than a big pile of underpants.

SECTION 4

LEVELING UP— ADVANCE IN THE GAME OF LIFE

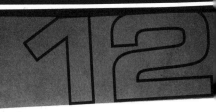

DEFINE YOUR LEVEL STRUCTURE

DO NOT GO GENTLE INTO THAT GOOD NIGHT,
OLD AGE SHOULD BURN AND RAVE AT CLOSE OF DAY;
RAGE, RAGE AGAINST THE DYING OF THE LIGHT.

—DYLAN THOMAS

Now that we're firmly immersed in the supernatural world portion of the Hero's Journey, it's time to start progressing through it by completing missions and tasks. If you've ever played *Destiny*, *Diablo*, or *EverQuest*, or even games like *Call of Duty*, you know leveling systems are beyond addicting. You'll play a game far after it's stopped being fun simply because there's the possibility of an increased level, a new achievement, or additional item. That's why you'll spend five hours killing rats just to get to the next level, as you'll then unlock a new sword or spell that gives you a chance to gain . . . yup, another level.

These leveling systems are designed specifically with human behavioral psychology in mind. As I told you earlier in the book, our brains love progress, and we love to be rewarded when we make progress. It's the same psychology behind why we feel good when somebody likes the photos we post to Facebook: we take an action, and we are rewarded for it. What's going on here? When these activities take place, our brains release dopamine, which makes us feel better and more accomplished. And then we chase that feeling. In fact, our brains can actually create new pathways with each repeated cue and reward.

Once we understand this process, it becomes our responsibility to use it for good rather than for evil. Although I don't play games like *EverQuest* very often anymore due to the time commitment they require and to my own admitted addiction to these types of games, I am still addicted to progress and leveling up. I just do it in real life now.

I want you to think again about those great games with fantastic leveling systems and what you can learn from them as you begin to make progress on the list of quests you've created. You don't jump from Level 1 to Level 50, right? You go from Level 1 to Level 2, to Level 3, and so on. There's a very clear progression from Zero to Hero, newbie to badass. On top of that, the challenges are presented in such a way that you are always incrementally pushing yourself just a bit more, stretching to fight bad guys just slightly better than you are. If you were to attack a Level 40 dragon when you're Level 5, you're going to get your ass kicked. However, after you've built up your character to Level 50, and are equipped with the most powerful weapon in the game, you're going to crush that dragon like a fly.

This is all possible thanks to solid game mechanics that build your experience and confidence as you move steadily up the ranks of the leveling system. So, how can we apply these rules and mechanics to our lives? By taking that list of quests and accomplishments and things we listed in the previous chapter, and seeing if we can break them down into smaller, bite-sized pieces or micro-levels and mini-quests. Think of each big quest on your list as a series of tiny, incremental quests. If we can create 10 steps to mastery of a skill, then we can focus our energy on simply putting one foot in front of the other and the process will take care of itself.

Let me give you some examples:

* Do you want to someday travel around the world but have never left your home state? That can be daunting, so why not start with a trip across state lines or go on an adventure in a different part of your country to give you the confidence to take the next step? I traveled to Peru with my buddy, Cash, to give me confidence and momentum to eventually book my solo around-the-world adventure.

* Do you want to become a black belt in karate, but you're overweight, stuck on the couch, and have never thrown a punch in your life? Start by committing to a workout routine and nutritional plan for a month or two to lose a few pounds and give yourself the confidence to sign up for a martial arts class.

* Do you want to start your own company but are stuck at a dead-end job? Spend the $10 to register a domain and start a website today, and go take out a book from the library on building a small business (or check the "Resources of The Rebellion" section at the back of this book for my tips on doing so!), and commit to working on that company for just 15 minutes a day.

In each of the examples above, take the smaller, more approachable, easier-to-accomplish item first so you can cross it off your list. Then take a closer look at the list to see if you can reorganize those specific quests in order of difficulty, along with any other organizational tactic you want to employ. I went with categories for mine, but your quests might be completely focused around one very specific type of category. If your game happens to be like *Rock Band*, for example, all of your quests might be music focused. That's fine.

Depending on how nerdy you want to get with this, you can assign different point values to your different quests based on their respective difficulty. I chose to keep my game relatively simple: each quest is worth 5, 10, or 20 experience points, and

100 experience points for every master quest completed. If you build your list on LevelUpYourLife.com, you can assign point values to the leveling system quite easily, and even break down your quest into mini-quests to make achieving progress less daunting.

SELECT YOUR FIRST QUEST AND GET STARTED

Remember, this is a lifelong journey, and we're going to take it step by step to crush one quest at a time and build momentum. So, don't worry about being able to accomplish the higher-difficulty items at the end of your quest just yet. Just as you can't expect to slay dragons when you're in the newbie zone, you shouldn't expect to win boss battles or cross every quest off your list just two weeks after starting out.

Tolkien's Boromir was wrong when he argued, "One does not simply walk into Mordor." That's actually exactly how you get to Mordor: one step at a time! It's the same technique I've employed to conquer this master quest of writing a book: one word at a time! And it's the same way you're going to start leveling up: one quest, one step, one day at a time.

I want you to take that first step now. Select the quest on your list that is the easiest for you to get started on. Pick one tiny portion of that quest that you can accomplish within the next 15 minutes—a portion that gets you one step closer to completing that item, and then do it. Right now. It needs to be something specific, actionable, and that brings you a step closer to completing the quest.

I'll wait.

I want you to commit to working on that quest for just 15 minutes every day. That might mean spending 15 minutes working on a blog post, or 15 minutes of exercise, or of learning to cook a healthier meal, or 15 minutes researching your first trip. All I want is 15 minutes. And remember, "I don't have time" no longer applies!

Let me give you a personal example. While writing this book, I decided I also wanted to learn to play the fiddle because why the hell not? I love Irish music, and one of my favorite bands is Gaelic Storm. I enjoyed my time in Ireland, and it just looked like a damn fun instrument to play. So, I searched "violin/fiddle lessons + Nashville," and found a violin studio that offers lessons for $30 an hour and will rent me a nice violin for only $20 a month! Jackpot! Now, "learn the violin" is a very broad goal, so I split it into a few mini-quests and a boss battle:

* **Level 1:** Commit to one violin lesson per week, and practice 15 minutes per day for six months. (100 exp)

* **Level 2:** Relearn how to read sheet music and complete *Celtic Fiddle Tunes* by Craig Duncan. (20 exp)

* **Level 3:** Learn to play "Concerning Hobbits" from *The Fellowship of the Ring* on the violin. (20 exp)

* **Level 4:** Sit and play the fiddle for 30 minutes with other musicians. (50 exp)

* **Level 5:** Learn to play "Promontory" from *The Last of the Mohicans* on the violin. (50 exp)

* **BOSS BATTLE:** Sit and play the fiddle for 30 minutes in a pub in Ireland. (100 exp)

When I started to play the violin, I struggled with getting myself to practice every day because the concept of practicing for an hour every day overwhelmed me. So, after failing for a while, I bought a violin stand. I did this so the violin would always be in tune, ready to be played, and in my line of sight when I walked in my apartment. Then I lowered my quest commitment to 15 minutes each day total. The result was that I started practicing daily, and often ended up putting in an hour or more of practice in 5-minute chunks spread throughout the day. In simplifying the quest, I made more progress in one month than I had made in the previous three.

/ CONTINUED ON PAGE 120 /

REBEL HERO

★ ★ ★ ★ ★ ★

NAME: Goran Dimic   AGE: 34

HOMETOWN: Zagreb, Croatia

I was thrilled to find Nerd Fitness and apply "gamification" to my life. I have been practicing several different forms of martial arts since I was seven years old. I have never considered myself to be a sporty guy, I just really loved Bruce Lee's awesome moves and mysterious secrets of the ninja. And that love has followed me for all my life, and still does. When I was in school, high school, even college, I always had time to go to regular practices, even hold my own classes.

I got a degree in preschool education, and went to get a job. But as I got a job, I realized that I have to stretch regularly and keep my body in swell shape because my body is my primary tool. Trips to the regular gym seemed so boring, and hard-core full contact sparring was out of the question—I just couldn't show up in a kindergarten where I work looking like a member of the Fight Club. So, as I said in the beginning, I've found Nerd Fitness, and the concept of gamification, and it rocked my world. Instead of run, I'd go on quests. Instead of rock climbing, I'd be planting/removing traps. I started making small scenarios and started playing with those ideas.

For instance: The X Quest. To achieve X (cinema night), I had to complete mission A: collect a flame sphere (do body weight exercises), mission B: scout the tower of shadow (go on a 20 minute light jog), and C: purify the temple of earth (clean up house, top to bottom). Complete missions in a time period of 1 week, each 3 times. So, that gives us the equation

SPOTLIGHT

DAY JOB: *Kindergarten Teacher*

ALTER EGO: *Gogor, the Hidden Master* **CLASS:** *Monk*

of: 3xA + 3xB + 3xC = X . First of all, it felt good to role-play this stuff, noting down the successes/finished missions, getting closer to unlocking the achievement. I felt good, because I was working out and had fun at the same time. It was good, because it made my fiancee (now wife) happy to see our little place, the temple of earth, shine and be spotless clean. And it was good, because it filled me with a sense of achievement.

The more I did it, the more I discovered how things can be "gamified." Achievements like: Designated Driver unlocked—as I did 50 drives for my nearest and dearest. Or my favorite: Iron Fist—for the first 200 knuckle push-ups that I did. I made my own handbook of favorite workouts, advices, and food recipes. I made my Epic Quest list of things to do. I use these concepts in my work, teaching a whole lot of positive stuff to kids. I'm doing more stuff easier because of it. By all means, that does not mean I don't fail every once in a while. I screw up, I make mistakes. But now, I'm smarter when facing "the next boss level" in life. Some say it's silly. But, hey—it works. It gives results; it makes me healthy and happy, makes life just more juicy and awesome to live.

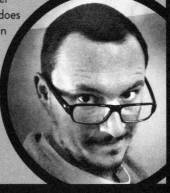

I won't be sitting in on any Irish jam sessions any time soon, but I had to start somewhere. I'm now a few months into my lessons, getting much better, and I'm having an absolute blast with it! I've even started to learn "Concerning Hobbits" (watch my progress at LevelUpYourLife.com).

Here's another example: let's say you also wanted to learn French. "Learn French" isn't specific enough; since that's a goal that's incredibly daunting let's break it down into a few levels:

* **Level 1:** Take one hour of French lessons twice a week for six months. (20 exp)
* **Level 2:** Practice for 20 minutes per day for six months. (20 exp)
* **Level 3:** Memorize the 100 most commonly spoken words in the French language. (20 exp)
* **Level 4:** Have a 30-minute conversation in French only with a native French speaker on Skype. (20 exp)
* **Level 5:** Save up enough money for a trip to France by 2020. (20 exp)
* **BOSS BATTLE:** Travel to France and spend one day only speaking French the entire day. (100 exp)

If you're somebody who wants to learn a new language, there's nothing stopping you from starting on that quest right now. I just took a break from writing this book to research French lessons and tracked down three native-speaking teachers on iTalki.com who will teach an hour lesson for less than $20 USD. Not bad!

These are a few basic examples, but they should help get you started. Remember, pick a quest, break it into teeny tiny levels, and spend 15 minutes completing the first mini quest. Incrementally, bit by bit, you'll move closer to mastery or completion of your main quest.

BE R.A.A.D: REEVALUATE, ADJUST, ADAPT, AND DOMINATE

We are on a journey, and sometimes journeys change. Maybe we've created a list of 50 quests, and we've come to learn that they are way too intimidating or difficult for us to get started. Or maybe we've gone there and back again, and determined that the quests we've set up are too easy. Each time we complete a quest or mission, or we go out and come back from a journey, we've learned something about ourselves, we've transformed a bit, and so we can evaluate how things have gone.

When we can objectively see how things have gone, we can then adjust our strategy for future quests or missions. That's why it's important to constantly evaluate and re-evaluate progress; that's how we grow. I encourage you to use a website or journal (or LevelUpYourLife.com) to track your journey. The path isn't always clear, but the fortune favors the bold and you can always course-correct along the way.

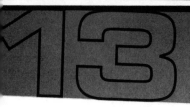

CONQUER BOSS BATTLES AND FIND TREASURE CHESTS

IT IS BY GOING DOWN INTO THE ABYSS THAT WE RECOVER THE TREASURES OF LIFE. WHERE YOU STUMBLE, THERE LIES YOUR TREASURE.

—JOSEPH CAMPBELL

Without making ourselves accountable to our goals, we have little incentive or impetus to succeed in achieving them. Think about a video game in which you can't die and you can't lose and you can get away with whatever you want. Sure, it might be fun to run around in "god mode" for a while, but once you remove the accountability factor of dying, the game ceases to be challenging. Conversely, take a game in which dying can be a huge detriment to making progress, and I bet you play that game with a lot more care and attention.

For example, playing *Diablo* in "Hardcore mode" means that deaths are permanent and you need to start over with a new character if you want to continue. It increases the challenge and fosters such a high level of dedication that gamers take the utmost care with each action and every battle.

It's with this same attitude that you will need to approach the idea of accountability in your Game of Life. Without establishing some sort of accountability when building new habits, tackling new activities, or engaging in new missions, you'll struggle to get started or fail to even get through your first few weeks of questing.

On the Hero's Journey, the hero reaches the innermost cave and faces enemies that challenge him to his very core. In video games, we face boss battles that test everything we've learned in the game up to that point. In life, accountability means the failure to complete a quest comes at a cost.

For example, let's say you decide you want to train for a marathon. If you skip your workout today, nothing much happens unless you make yourself accountable. You get to not only skip the run you weren't looking forward to, but also spend your time sitting on the couch playing *Call of Duty*. There's no negative consequence to your actions (or lack thereof) besides not getting fitter, which is tough to gauge day-to-day.

However, if the same skipped workout automatically triggered a $100 transfer from your checking account into the political campaign fund of a candidate you despise, you'd probably get off your ass and go, "Ugh, fine, I'll just do the damn thing." Congratulations, you just introduced a level of accountability to your leveling system! Ultimately, what you're doing here is increasing the negative consequence of skipping the life-changing activity until it's greater than the perceived "pain" of actually completing it. In doing this, you're essentially adding a boss battle to your quest that will kick your ass unless you follow through with your training.

I have a really good friend named Chris St. James ("Saint" for short) who I've known since the fourth grade. We played sports and video games together all through grade school, high school, and then virtually through college and beyond. After college he packed on a bunch of weight while working a desk job, and after struggling to lose it for years he finally managed to drop a crazy amount of weight and eventually got to 9 percent body fat. How was he able to break through and crush his weight-loss goal months ahead of schedule? By introducing accountability.

I'll never forget the day: Saint called me in a panic and said, "I've made a huge mistake." My first thought was, "Do I need to bail you out of jail?" Fortunately, that wasn't the issue. Saint told me he'd bet a friend he could get to 9 percent body fat before his wedding, six months down the road, or he would owe his friend $500. Because money was tight for Saint at the time, the thought of losing $500 was so terrifying that it motivated him to dedicate himself fully to achieving his goal. By agreeing to the wager, Saint introduced two important elements to his game: He added both an accountability system and a deadline, and he rose to the challenge. You can see Saint's photos and story at LevelUpYourLife.com.

Benny Lewis, creator of FluentIn3Months.com, set a target goal of learning a new language to the point of conversational fluency every time he visited a new country. Because tourist visas generally expire after three months, he always has a very real deadline for the achievement of his goal. This was an aggressive timeline, but because it was also very specific he knew exactly what needed to be done week-to-week, day-to-day, in order to reach his goal. Although Benny spoke only English until he was in his early twenties, he's now conversationally fluent in eight languages!

The more specific you can be with the level of accountability you can add to a quest you're working on, the more likely you'll be to follow through with the action and succeed. Want to run more? Sign up with friends for a half-marathon that's six months down the road, and prepay for it. Even if you've never run a day in your life, you'll now be able to reverse-engineer your training schedule so you'll be on pace to run that half marathon six months down the road or else face the ridicule of your friends. Suddenly, "I want to run more" will become "I will run the Runner's World Half Marathon in Bethlehem, Pennsylvania, in October." Not only do you have a very real deadline, but you have a questing party, too—your friends are also training and can help keep you accountable on the days you feel like skipping. Win!

If you want to visit a foreign country and learn its language, pick a date in the future for your trip and, if possible, book the trip, put down a deposit, or start saving for it right away. Resolve that in [insert month] you will visit [insert country] and spend an entire day there conversing only in [insert language of that country]. That takes a vague goal like, "I want to travel," or "I'd like to learn a new language," and makes it way more specific, concrete, and real. Now, with money on the line and a date set, you'll have to start taking language lessons or you'll end up flying overseas and struggling to communicate.

Would you like to build a new business or write a book but can't get yourself to actually take action? Just add accountability. To motivate myself to write articles ahead of schedule for Nerd Fitness, I have given $500 to Team Nerd Fitness member Staci. If I miss an article deadline, she's been instructed to donate $50 to the Westboro Baptist Church. Because it sickens me to donate my hard-earned money to a cause I don't believe in, I now have a built-in motivation to get my work done instead of slacking off. To date, exactly $0 has been donated.

THE POWER OF REWARDS

Holding oneself accountable isn't easy. It requires grit, perseverance, and stamina. How do the world's best adventurers hold themselves accountable to fulfilling their hero's destiny and completing their quests? By introducing powerful rewards to energize them along the way, in addition to the accountability we just discussed.

/ CONTINUED ON PAGE 128 /

REBEL HERO

★ ★ ★ ★ ★ ★

NAME: Natascha Kotte   **AGE:** 22

HOMETOWN: Parañaque, Philippines

It started when I got an article from the Nerd Fitness Rebellion about 20 seconds of courage (which is a power-up explained later in this book!). I've been using the hell out of it ever since. That day, I decided to try out this new power-up and sign myself up for a college ballroom dancing class.

It was one of the best things I could have done for myself even though I was terrified and didn't speak to anyone in class for the first half of the semester. Learning ballroom dancing at first is exactly like the sweetness of working a skill tree in a role playing game and grinding until I was at a high enough level to move on to the next.

Once I realized that I could gamify the rest of my world, that there was more to life than being in a rut, I shot outwards in all directions I could think of and just went for everything. I quit my college bookstore job and applied to become a lab assistant. I now get to work in my major and it's the best job on campus. I asked out my studio instructor out for lunch last year. We're still together and met each other's respective families.

I spent the summer working on my social and dance skill trees in Las Vegas: dancing every night to live music and learning to hang out and kick back with great performers. I've even decided to try out a leadership quest and I am now the

SPOTLIGHT

DAY JOB: *R&D Microbiologist*

ALTER EGO: *Tash, the Desert Munchkin* **CLASS:** *Druid*

president of the UNLV American Chemical Society student chapter.

Now, it hasn't been the smoothest of roads. I went from a terrified novice hiding in the back of ballroom class to gliding out onto the competition floor for the first time only to trip over my own feet. That's just one of the many things that would have sent me scuttling back to my cave if I didn't have the mindset I do now. I work with the perspective now that life has become one big game for me and it's only going to get better as I level up. Sometimes I may trip, but that doesn't mean I have to whack the reset button and start all over again in the training fields.

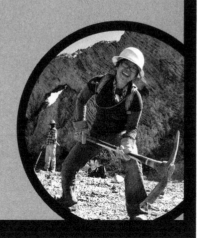

When I think about the link between rewards and accountability, my brain immediately goes to The Legend of Zelda series. By the time you've completed a dungeon level in a Legend of Zelda game, you'll have received a heart container (upping your health meter), a piece of the Triforce (which you need put back together in order to succeed), and treasure chests that contain a new weapon or item that allows you to advance further in the game.

If you've ever seen a science experiment in which a rat or monkey hits a button or solves a puzzle and is rewarded with food, then you know a reward can be very powerful, especially when starting out. While it would be nice to tell ourselves that the reward of getting healthy should be enough to get us to work out, or that the reward of financial freedom is enough to get us to start saving, our brains don't work that way. In most cases, the allure of immediate gratification on our lizard brains is so strong that we sabotage our efforts to level up our lives in the long term in exchange for happiness in the short term. If given the choice:

* ✳ "Sugar makes my brain happy so I'm going to eat this donut" will win out over: "Six months from now I'm going to fit into smaller clothes."

* ✳ "Playing *Diablo* for three hours makes me happy" will win out over: "If I work on this book proposal, I can get a book deal and publish a book two years from now."

* ✳ "Checking my phone to see Facebook updates makes me happy" will win out over: "If I become more productive at work, I can get a raise or go home early and spend more time with my family."

But, just as we needed to increase the consequences for skipping the activities that enable us to actually complete our quests, so too can we reward ourselves for following through with the healthier or more productive behavior.

However, we're not going to follow the typical reward path most people follow. Have you ever heard someone say something like, "I worked out today, so I earned this pint of ice cream"? Or "I had a tough day at work, so I earned this six pack of Duff Beer?" Or "I followed through with my goals this week, so I get to have [activity with negative end result]"? In each of those instances, we're rewarding ourselves for completing a positive activity with something that sends us back one or two steps. So instead of rewarding ourselves with crap that doesn't help us in the long run, we're going to instead reward ourselves with things that contribute meaningfully toward helping us achieve our overarching goals. We'll call these rewards "treasure chests." As you're building your reward system around the quest you're currently working on, see if there's a way you can reward yourself with a treasure chest that has lasting impact on or benefit to your game. For example:

* Once you lose 50 pounds, reward yourself with new workout clothes; you'll feel better about yourself and actually WANT to go to the gym more.
* Once you've completed your first 5K, treat yourself to a new pair of running shoes that will encourage you to run more.
* Once you've completed the first draft of your book manuscript, take a trip to a writer's conference that will inspire you to keep writing.
* Once you complete a month worth of language learning, buy yourself a new movie or book in that language that will encourage you to want to further your studies.

These rewards, when combined with a deadline and accountability, can be the difference between achieving success and struggling through yet another year in which you talk a big game but never make any real changes. When you are just getting started with learning new skills or trying to build new habits to replace unhealthy ones, rewards and accountability can both be incredibly powerful motivators to help us step on the gas and get moving.

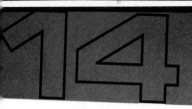

PERSEVERE IN THE FACE OF OBSTACLES AND ORDEALS

MOTIVATION IS WHAT GETS YOU STARTED.
HABIT IS WHAT KEEPS YOU GOING.   —JIM ROHN

No hero makes it through his or her journey without encountering trouble. And thank goodness. Think of how boring that story would be! Every great story includes obstacles the hero must overcome: the greater the challenge the greater the reward. The question is, how will you handle these challenges as you attempt to complete the quest or mission before you? Will you look at them as opportunities to grow and advance—to prove to yourself that you are capable of leveling up—or will you look at them as brick walls that halt your progress? It all comes down to your attitude and your strategy for attacking the obstacle.

Rewards and accountability can only take us so far. If we truly want to achieve long-term success, we first need to understand how willpower works, to cultivate discipline, and to get ourselves into the flow as often possible.

If you've always wanted to write a book but instead sit around until you're motivated to get started (or waiting for inspiration to strike), that book will never get written. If you struggle each month to save money to put toward a fun adventure, you're relying too much on willpower to get things done! I'm here to tell you the problem isn't that you lack willpower or that you don't have enough motivation. The problem is that willpower is a finite resource, and motivation is fleeting. If we are going to succeed, we need to radically adjust how we attack our problems and conquer the missions we've created for ourselves.

If you've ever said, "Why can't I get myself to exercise?" or "I can't stop myself when I eat poorly," or "I would love to travel, but I can't get myself to save money," then you are a victim of a depleted willpower resource. Believe it or not, as the following study points out, your willpower can behave exactly like your hit points (HP) in a video game:

In a study at Case Western Reserve University, subjects were split into two groups and presented with both fresh-baked cookies and radishes. One group could eat cookies or radishes and the other group was ONLY allowed to eat radishes. Afterward, both groups were given an impossible maze to solve. The ones who had to restrain themselves from eating cookies gave up more than TWICE as fast as the group that had been allowed to eat cookies.

Think of the three most common ways you tend to die when playing a game. You attack a bad guy who's too powerful; you attack too many bad guys at once; or you start an attack before you've fully recovered from your last attack.

Here in real life, things aren't much different; just replace "hit points" with "willpower":

1. **Attack a bad guy who's too powerful**

   If you haven't exercised in a decade and try to run a marathon, you'll probably collapse five minutes into the race. If you decide you want to learn French and you immediately sign up for 10 hours of French lessons, you might give up before you even get started because you're so intimidated.

2. **Attack too many bad guys at once**

   When playing an RPG, you don't run into a room full of enemies and attack all of them at once like the infamous Leeroy Jenkins in *World of Warcraft*; you're going to get overwhelmed and get your ass kicked. Instead, you pick them off one by one by one, increasing your chances of survival by approximately 132.33 percent (repeating, of course). This is why most New Year's resolution makers fail miserably within two weeks—they try to make twenty changes at once and quickly get overwhelmed!

3. **Attack before you're fully recovered**

   Any time you get into a battle, you're probably going to lose some health. If you take the time to recover, your health will most likely return to 100 percent by the next battle. However, if you fight 10 battles in a row without any rest, you can run into some trouble. The next battle might be against some super-easy bad guy, but could promptly result in a "game over" simply because you're down to a single heart container! After spending all day taxing your body with work and difficult decisions, coming home and bypassing the couch, your Xbox, and a freezer full of ice cream to get changed and start exercising is going to be incredibly difficult. That's because you're not giving your willpower points a chance to recharge!

If willpower is a finite resource, then you might be wondering what sort of things deplete it, and if there's a way to replenish it. As I learned from Charles Duhigg's book, *The Power of*

Habit, our bodies will do everything possible to be more efficient, opting in every situation to use less willpower and choose the path of least resistance. Because we are creatures of habit, we can look to our current habits to see what happens when our bodies operate on autopilot, as that's exactly how we got to where we are. We've repeated certain activities—good or bad—so many times our brains have learned to complete them almost automatically. Whenever we try to build new habits (exercising, flossing, spending less money, getting off the couch and adventuring), our brains have to work a little extra because we're focusing on a new action rather than passively completing a routine that has become habit.

How do we develop a new action into an automatic habit? By making sure the new action is both achievable and repeatable. That's why in the previous chapter I asked you to pick a single quest, select a tiny part of it that you could accomplish immediately, and check off a box that says, "I'm awesome—I completed part of my quest today." If you aren't making progress on a quest, just break it down into even smaller pieces (or mini-quests) so you have no choice but to make progress. To quote the film *The Patriot:* "Aim small, miss small." If you don't bite off more than you can chew, you won't get overwhelmed, and your odds of success will increase.

Here are a few of my favorite examples:

* If you want to exercise five days a week, start by going for a walk for five minutes each morning. No more than five minutes. And then go for a freaking walk, right now.

* If you want to learn a new language, spend just 10 minutes per day this week reviewing flash cards or talking to somebody. Ten minutes, tops.

* If you want to start a blog, set a goal of writing just 300 words per day at the start. Then focus only on writing those 300 words each morning before you do anything else. If that sounds like too much, lower the daily word count to 100!

Remember, the goal here is to commit to doing just a little bit each day. Make it something you can measure, but something you commit to! Something you can cross off a list and say: "I did this today." The benefits or results of this one activity might not make itself apparent after a day or so, or maybe even a week. After all, we're asking you to pick the smallest change possible so you have no choice but to complete it. You might even be looking at this and saying, "Steve this is too simple, I'm capable of doing more than this."

That's the point!

The benefits of a single day spent working on your current quest pale in comparison to the bigger reason why you're doing this: to prove to yourself that you can make progress, and that working on a quest daily can become a new habit for you—a new normal. You are taking steps to proving to yourself that the destiny you laid out for yourself earlier in the book is possible to realize; that life at Level 50 can and will happen with enough forward progress. It's these tiny incremental steps, mini boss battles, and small victories on our quests that give us a chance to actually succeed on a larger scale.

UPGRADE YOUR BATCAVE

You know how I said we are creatures of habit? It turns out we are products of our environment as well.

The locations where you live, work, and play influence your behavior far more than you probably realize. Your brain is constantly taking stock of what's around you and reacting to what you see. Depending on how you have acted in the past, if you visit Facebook.com, your brain might think, "I get Likes and fun and happiness when I log on to Facebook." When you see your comfy couch and giant TV, your brain might say, "I get hours of entertainment here." Reactions like these have been reinforced through hundreds of repetitions. Just as driving a car has become, through repetition, something you can do without much thought, so too are all the things your brain thinks when you complete the previous activities. Every time you restrain yourself from doing those things—or you choose instead to do something healthier, better, or more adventurous—you have to use willpower and brainpower to make things happen. And then, over time, those deliberate actions become automatic habits. Think about it this way:

If you want to go for a run when you get home from work (after you've already used up all your willpower and decision-making brainpower during the workday), you need to walk past that comfy couch, your video game systems, and your refrigerator (FOOD! HAPPY!). Then you have to walk into your bedroom, change into your workout clothes, lace up your shoes, and walk past all of those amazing distractions all over again on your way out the door.

If you want to become more productive at work, you have to force yourself to stop checking Facebook, Twitter, Instagram, ESPN, Gmail, and other addictive sites and apps 100+ times a day. You have to consistently remind and restrict your brain to say: "To hell with you, amazing time-wasting websites and apps that provide me with instant gratification and external validation, I'm going to focus on the task at hand!" That's like trying to type a report about 16th-century agrarian economics in the middle of Times Square, while people in panda costumes play the bagpipes next to you. Good luck getting *that* paper done, pal!

In order for us to stop depleting our willpower and letting decision fatigue derail our goals of world domination and adventure, we need to build a better Batcave. You don't need to build a Batmobile, and you don't need to put on a costume (unless you want to—I'd never knock a hero for putting on a costume). What I simply mean is that Bruce Wayne spends a lot of his time in his Batcave leveling up his life, and the Batcave is specifically designed to help him defeat criminals. I want you to start doing the same thing with your life.

Think about the three environments in which you spend most of your time: your home, your car, and your office. The more small adjustments you can make to those environments—adjustments that serve to decrease the number of steps between you and building a good habit and increase the number of steps between you and a bad habit—the less you'll have to rely on willpower. As I read in a Quora thread when somebody asked the question "How do I get motivated?": "F%*k motivation. Instead, cultivate discipline."

It starts by building a Batcave that sets you up to succeed.

ADD STEPS BETWEEN YOU AND BAD HABITS

Here's an example of how I adjusted my own Batcave over the past year. First, I noticed I was spending way too much time watching TV and not enough time writing this book. I continued to tell myself I didn't have time, when in reality I had plenty of time—I was simply spending it inefficiently. I needed to start working smarter, not harder. So I canceled my cable. Suddenly, with nothing on television to distract me, I had one extra step between me and wasting time. And after a few days, I didn't miss it.

Say you are trying to save more money for a trip, but you consistently find yourself buying junk food or digging yourself further into credit card debt. Can you automate your finances so that a few bucks are pulled from your paycheck automatically into a separate account before you even know it's missing?

Take some time right now to identify some of the bad habits you already have, and then think of steps you can add between you and indulging those habits. The harder you make it on yourself to fall back into a bad habit, the better. If that means putting a combination lock on your cookie jar (or, even better, throwing the jar away), cutting your cable like I did, or blocking distracting websites during work hours, so be it.

REMOVE STEPS BETWEEN YOU AND GOOD HABITS

It's been said that it's twice as tough to break a bad habit than it is to build a new habit, so let's switch our focus to something you want to do but can't get yourself to do consistently. By removing steps between you and the new skill you're trying to develop, the more likely you'll be to make learning that skill a habit.

For example, let's say you've always wanted to read more but never seem to find the time to do it. Why not minimize the steps between you and "I finished a book"? Download the Amazon Kindle app on your phone, pick up an actual Kindle, and bring it with you everywhere. You can read a page or two while waiting for the bus or train, while in line getting lunch, or while on your designated coffee break. This technique of reading whenever I have a few free minutes allows me to get through way more books than I ever have in the past.

James Clear of JamesClear.com started flossing by buying floss picks and putting them in the middle of the vanity in his bathroom, telling himself he only had to floss one tooth every day. That's it. Of course, once he flossed one tooth, he was far more inclined to floss the others, and now he's sure to get a clean bill of oral health from his dentist!

I want you to start adjusting your Batcave and set yourself up for success, too. Identify the places you spend the most time, and make small changes to those environments to minimize the amount of willpower required to stay on target.

If you watch too much TV, consider canceling your cable. Not only will it save you roughly $80+ dollars a month (which you can automatically add to a savings account for future adventures), but it'll save you from hours of watching stupid crap! If there are shows you love to watch—*The Walking Dead, Game of Thrones,* and so forth—spend the $2 per episode on those individual shows.

If you want to run or exercise every morning, sleep in your running clothes! Place your alarm clock across the room from your bed, with your shoes right next to it and a glass of water. Make the alarm sound as annoying as possible, hop out of bed, quickly put your running shoes on, and get it done. If you want to exercise after work, pack your gym bag the night before and leave it by your front door so you never forget it on your way out in the morning. Don't even give yourself the option of coming home before going to work out.

If you're the type of person who struggles with getting *anything* done after work, then try getting those important adventure-life-building tasks done before you go to work by getting up earlier. Don't wait for decision fatigue and willpower to take over your life.

I've come to learn that success, adventure, happiness, and even greatness aren't things we're born with—in fact, they aren't even the end goal. Instead they are things that can be learned, habits that can be built, and the byproducts of our efforts to build our lives around our quests. If you're serious about leveling up your life, start by furiously eliminating the unimportant parts of your life to free you up for what truly is important. With each change, we get a tiny bit more likely to achieve what we're after: building momentum and getting into the flow.

BECOME AN UNSTOPPABLE FORCE OF AWESOME

AN OBJECT AT REST STAYS AT REST, AND AN OBJECT IN MOTION STAYS IN MOTION WITH THE SAME SPEED AND IN THE SAME DIRECTION UNLESS ACTED UPON BY AN UNBALANCED FORCE. —SIR ISAAC NEWTON (PARAPHRASED)

Imagine that you are Bowser, the incredibly large (and strong) King Koopa in the Mario Kart series. Due to Bowser's immense size, you have a very fast top speed, but rather poor acceleration. When you step on the gas pedal, it takes a tremendous amount of effort to get your kart to move even an inch. However, if you continue to hammer on that pedal, your kart will start to move faster and faster until you reach top speed. At this point, even a slight touch of the gas will allow your kart to continue moving forward, due to inertia and momentum (thank you, science!).

When you are beginning your quest, you are like Bowser at the starting line. We need to step on the gas and get you moving, but it takes a lot of effort as we have a lot of inertia to overcome in order to get started. This is especially true if you're living in your mom's basement, you're overweight, or you don't have a great job. In the game, it's Bowser's size that gives him slow acceleration. For us in real life, it's our bad habits, obligations, and struggles with focus and discipline that we need to overcome.

I want you to think of every single tiny step forward on each quest as being another second with your foot on the gas pedal. We spent Chapter 13 determining our future identity as a world-changing superhero; we need to now prove to ourselves consistently that we are getting closer and closer to our goal. It's tough going at first, but we have to start somewhere, and each tiny victory makes it more and more likely that we'll prove to ourselves that we can change.

Every time we experience a small win or a quest success, we are building up momentum, and telling that self-limiting belief in our brain that says "I suck!" that it's wrong. That might be tough to picture, so I took the liberty of creating this handy graphic for you below.

Imagine you're pushing the giant rock like in the graphic below. At first, the rock requires a TON of effort to move (there's a lot of "I suck" to overcome!), but as you earn small win after small win, the slope gets more gradual, the "I win!" starts to happen more often, and eventually less and less effort is required to

Overcoming Self-Limiting Beliefs

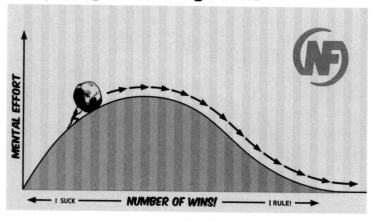

reinforce your positive behavior and build more confidence. In essence, your self-limiting belief gets beat up and replaced by a positive self-fulfilling prophecy!

Just like in Mario Kart, you only have to continue to build momentum and drive super fast on a nice easy course with no distractions. Ha, just kidding. That game would be boring as hell, which is why the Mario Kart series has turtle shells, lightning bolts, banana peels, bombs, and so on mucking up the roadway: it keeps things interesting. Life is loaded with obstacles, too; some of which can be avoided with clever driving, while others can be powered through.

THE FUEL FOR DRIVE

When I first started working out 14 years ago, I did it because I was sick of being the weak, scrawny kid. I wanted to build muscles and get big and strong so I could try to make the high school basketball team (this was after I got cut—mostly because I sucked!). My goals were very externally focused: "If I work out, then I will build muscle and get better at sports and look better and thus have more confidence and maybe finally get a date." I was so focused on the scale and how I looked in the mirror that I based a lot of my self-worth on that outward appearance. I had a deadline ("basketball tryouts") and accountability—although my brother had graduated the previous year, my friends were on the team and I wanted to join them. However, something funny happened while on my journey: I built the habit of exercise, and I fell in love with it.

These days, I've stopped counting calories and no longer freak out if I don't get enough protein each and every day. As a result of these changes, I'm now in the best shape of my life and feel more confident than ever! I don't go to the gym to exercise; I go to the gym because I truly enjoy my time there. I love the feeling of chalk on my hands and wrists as I set up for muscle-ups, an exercise I couldn't complete until recently. I love feeling like freaking Wolverine; my body's central nervous system is in berserker mode

(*CONTINUED ON PAGE 144*)

REBEL HERO

★ ★ ★ ★ ★ ★

NAME: Austin Smith   **AGE:** 25

HOMETOWN: Ames, IA

I am a combat veteran who struggles with depression and PTSD, so mental health is critical for me. To boot, I have minor back and knee problems from my service time. I have been working on identifying skills in my life that align with my interests so that I don't have to force myself to do them and that don't put me at too much risk for injury.

I try to find hidden workouts or benefits in nontraditional activities so that I can gamify them and level up. It's involved discovering and pursuing multiple skill trees, especially the following:

- Gardening—Even if it's a small space or window containers, it can be done!
- Cooking—More of it and with as little processed ingredients as possible. We've made serious cutbacks in the amount of eating out that we do.
- Livestock Handling—My wife and I have started to raise meat rabbits as a stepping stone into higher levels.
- Archery—It's downright fun, and is a great mental and physical workout. Especially with traditional equipment like my longbow, Serenity.
- Hunting—It works for exercise, mental health, and healthy diet. Don't underestimate the workout potential of bringing your dinner home over rough terrain!
- Crafting—I've been acquiring resources and tools to

SPOTLIGHT

DAY JOB: College Student

ALTER EGO: Liado   **CLASS:** Adventurer

begin learning how to tan and craft leather goods. Only failed attempts so far, but that can happen when you're a low level like me.

- Lore—Studying and immersing myself in nature, which is perfect for hiking and running outside of the city. It comes in handy when you can identify wild edibles to take home or snack on while on-the-go.

- Construction—Tinkering with minor stuff like rabbit structures and simple household furniture is a good relief from outside stress and keeps me moving and flexible. Doing all of these things has really been helping me in a myriad of ways.

Thanks to The Rebellion, I'm finding ways to improve not only my overall health but that of my wife's as well. We are always seeking new adventures. Our dreams require skills that neither of us were exposed to earlier in life, so we're making the effort to level up in preparation for our future. And The Rebellion has showed me well how to prepare for the challenges ahead.

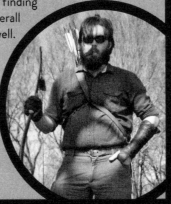

after setting a new personal best on deadlifts—moving closer to my epic quest goal of pulling 405 pounds. I love working on my handstands and experiencing that moment in which I'm in perfect balance upside down and time stops, my scatterbrained mind suddenly finding focus and repeating one phrase: "Don't move."

No matter how good or bad my day is going—no matter what's going on with my friends, business, or family—the gym is always there, challenging me to see if I'm a little bit better than I was last time.

I noticed something while reading the book *Drive*, by Dan Pink, and thinking about the people I've helped lose weight and get healthy through Nerd Fitness. In almost every single one of our success stories, there has been a recurring theme. People who have had lasting success and finally cracked the code have all, at one time or another, said: "I never thought I'd say this, but I actually look forward to exercising now."

Think about that previous statement for a second: these are people who most likely never exercised a day in their lives, were often 100+ pounds overweight, and generally despised exercising, but they all reached a point where they truly, genuinely look forward to the activity. This isn't just a new habit. They're fulfilling something deeply rooted within our DNA, something that craves exercise, physical activity, and adventure. We're designed to move and be active, to be curious about what's next or where we're going—it's just been lost in us because it's no longer a requirement for our survival like it was back in the Fred Flintstone days.

Luckily, what has been lost or missing can be found! It's like a switch is flipped. Suddenly, insurmountable challenges become conquerable. Positivity and "If I could do that, what else am I capable of?" become the rule, not the exception. It's an upward spiral. Success begets success, adventure encourages more of it, and travel inspires us to travel more. We fall in love with constant improvement—we get addicted to how it makes us feel. Drive becomes incredibly important to us and to the life quests we choose to undertake while assuming our heroic alter egos. This importance manifests in perhaps the most significant component of our life-quest gameplay: Flow, baby. Flow.

GAMEPLAY FLOW = GAMEPLAY MASTERY

As I pointed out back in Chapter 7 about happiness, we are at our most happy when we can get in the zone while performing a challenging or engaging activity. In nerd speak: you are having so much fun and are so immersed in the activity at hand that you lose track of time. Although I often find myself in the zone while playing specific video games, I try to target most of my flow on beneficial activities that improve my life!

Although the book *Drive* speaks about flow in terms of work, it can also apply to leveling up in our lives. How does that happen? Here are the three ways you can get yourself into flow:

1. **MASTERY:** Fall in love with consistent, marked improvement. If you can complete a new language quiz that was more difficult than last week's quiz, you're improving. If you are perfecting the art of the handstand and working on holding it for fractions of a second longer than before, you're getting stronger. As they say, "That which is measured gets improved."

2. **ENJOYMENT:** Do it because you enjoy it. If you lose track of time while running, cooking, doing yoga, reading, traveling, learning, playing piano, or rock climbing, you've found the activity that you need to spend more time doing! If you're lucky, you can find this in your job. But if instead you are forced to seek enjoyment in your spare time, you may need to eliminate unnecessary distractions in those hours in order to free up more time to pursue your passions.

3. **PURPOSE:** Be part of something bigger than yourself. I'm truly honored and proud to be part of The Rebellion. We have

a massive community of nerds, underdogs, desk jockeys, and average Joes and Jills, working hard at improving their lives in every facet. Whether you realize it or not, your journey and your quest for a better life are probably inspiring more people than you realize. The sooner you can get started with living a life that makes you happy, the sooner those around you will get inspired to do the same.

The more time you can spend every day in flow, the happier you will be—the challenge is to make sure you are targeting activities that reward you back with a leveled-up life! The more wins you can have every day, the more momentum you will build. We can start by constantly seeking little changes and improvements that show we're on the right path, and that will prove to us that we can get better at, and master, a subject, skill, or talent. It all starts with identifying the things we hope to accomplish, breaking those things into manageable levels, mini-quests, and missions, and making sure we set aside time for doing things purely out of enjoyment. Lastly, I want you to remember that you don't exist in a vacuum—you're part of a pretty special group of Rebels who are all trying to improve—and we need you fighting alongside us. We all want to live lives of adventure, lives that challenge us to become better people, to leave the world a better place, and to have stories we'll look back on with each other and say, "Remember the time we did that?"

This last point is crucial. Because life is a massively multiplayer game, we can use the same game mechanics and character archetypes from our favorite stories to help build our questing party.

Let's go looking for a group.

16

CHOOSE MULTIPLAYER MODE AND BUILD A LEGENDARY TEAM

44 WIZZY LOOKING FOR GROUP IN EVERFROST!
—MORPHOS NOVASTORM (MY CHARACTER IN EVERQUEST)

Remember that first time you jumped into an online game like *World of Warcraft*? Not only did you get to create a character and explore a new, mysterious, amazing world . . . but there were other ACTUAL people running around with you! Heck, they could even be people you knew in real life. Although this might seem old hat now, way back in the late 1990s it was a big deal.

I remember one particularly boring evening in which I was once again glued to my computer playing *EverQuest*. I was at the Wizard Spires in the Plains of North Karanas with my character

Morphos, and I saw this tiny dot in the distance slowly getting larger and larger. Eventually, this dot became a character, and I saw it was my good friend, Saint. Even though he lived 10 minutes down the road from me in real life, I was absolutely blown away at the fact that we could hang out and see each other in a game at the same time. We spent a good two hours typing "/dance" and laughing hysterically over our landline telephone—we just couldn't believe how far games had come.

This is why I fell in love with massively multiplayer online role-playing games (MMORPGs). I loved the idea of creating well-balanced groups of heroes, going on dungeon raids, treasure hunting, connecting with new people from all over the globe, and exploring locations I never could have explored alone. Unfortunately, all this behavior took place while I sat home alone at my computer, but that's okay! It made me realize that just as video games can succeed or fail based on their multiplayer component, so too can this MMORPG we call life. Yes, Life is a massively multiplayer game. And when you can spend more time surrounded by the people you love, or people who challenge you to be better, and less time surrounded by people who drag you down, your chances for happiness in the Game of Life are greatly improved. As Christopher McCandless, the main subject in the book/movie *Into the Wild*, tragically wrote before passing away: "Happiness is only real when shared."

Or, as researchers at Brigham Young University and the University of North Carolina at Chapel Hill discovered, those with poor social connections had on average 50 percent higher odds of death in the study's follow-up period (an average of 7.5 years) than people with more robust social ties. To put that in perspective, this mortality gap is as large as that between smokers and nonsmokers!

Now, thanks to the advance of social media, it's become much easier to "connect" with people without having to actually spend time with them in person, and this can be detrimental to our happiness: it's cool to connect with people via video games, but that isn't a substitute for real-life interaction and engagement. We can learn from how games use online multiplayer or local multiplayer to be more enjoyable, and then apply it to life.

It's important to bear in mind that the people you choose to join you in your game will have a significant impact on your adventure: just as playing with poor sports, complainers, and bums who make rude comments about your mother can ruin a video game experience, hanging out with chumps in real life can have the same impact.

On any Hero's Journey, when the hero enters into the unknown world, he or she will encounter—and must win over—allies, enemies, sidekicks, and guardians. These characters, such as in *The Fellowship of the Ring* or *The Avengers*, exist to advance the plot, shake things up, keep things interesting, and provide the hero with an opportunity to grow, adapt, and change.

Because we know willpower is fleeting and motivation is difficult to maintain long term, we need to not only build our environment in a way that sets us up for success but also to build a proper multiplayer experience. Luckily for you, I've gone ahead and done the legwork on how to build the perfect team. You just need to start recruiting the right members.

SURROUND YOURSELF WITH PEOPLE BETTER THAN YOU

Say you're playing a role-playing game and you get to team up with five other characters to go on quests for the evening. Which of the following two groups would you choose?

* **Group A:** Five characters who are all at lower levels than you, who rely on you for everything and aren't very good at the game. You constantly die, but you get to say you're the best of this terrible group.

* **Group B:** Five characters who are all at higher levels than you. They have epic skills, all play different classes, have

different play styles, constantly push to fight bad guys who are at higher levels than you, show you the ropes, and allow you to explore more locations than you could have explored in the past.

The answer is obvious, no? If given the choice, we'd all choose to be part of Group B. Think about how much more exciting it is when you join a group of higher-level people that you can learn from:

* You get to explore more dangerous and challenging places you wouldn't have been able to see otherwise.
* You kill dragons you would have never been able to slay.
* You level faster than you would have leveled if you went questing alone.
* You die far less often and get to have more fun.

If this is universally accepted behavior in games (looking to join the best), why do we allow ourselves to get stuck in crappy groups in real life? Why don't we constantly try to level up and group up with characters who are better than us? Those who push us to be better people? Who challenge us to try to keep up? It's time to level up our groups.

When we encounter the characters in a game who are better than everybody else, something important comes to mind: you're instantly inspired to play more. You know it took this guy days and days of questing, grinding, and dungeon crawling to get there, but if he can reach Level 50 and get all that cool stuff, so can you one day. In real life, the same can be true! When we surround ourselves with people who have had more success, who have traveled more, who have done the things we've always wanted to do, it can inspire, motivate, and encourage us to be better ourselves. Not only that, but these people show us exactly how to move up a few levels. Rather than saying, "Must be nice to be them," we can start saying, "Hey, if they can do it, so can I!"

In the book *Faster, Higher, Stronger*, author Mark McClusky, senior editor of *Wired* magazine, interviewed the director of sports development at USA Volleyball, John Kessel. Kessel explained that a disproportionate number of their best players were younger siblings. Why? Because: "The more you play against bigger kids, older kids, even adults, the better you become as an athlete." In laymen's terms: the more time you spend with people who are better, more successful, healthier, and happier than you, the types of decisions you make and the things you choose to do will be constantly influenced by those people. Just as more adventures present themselves to us when we begin to see life itself as an adventure, more group adventures pop up when we surround ourselves with people who feel that same way.

Let's start by identifying the types of people we want on our team, and the character archetypes with whom we want to group.

HOW TO BUILD AN ELITE MULTIPLAYER GROUP

The Jedi Order. The Avengers. The A-Team.

What do these groups all have in common? They are each comprised of unique individuals with special talents that help everybody else in the group get better (or stronger, or faster, or more badass). They are greater than the sum of their parts. Contrast this with a homogenous collection of Storm Trooper clones in which everybody has the same strengths and weaknesses.

Now, having an army of 1,000 Supermans (or Supermen?) would be pretty awesome right? Wrong! If we had 1,000 of them, it would still only take a wee bit of kryptonite to take them ALL down. However, when you have Superman AND Batman AND Wonder Woman AND yes, even Aquaman, suddenly picking apart the Justice League's weaknesses becomes far more difficult.

Long story short: Diversity rules! In games, in movies, in books, and in our lives, having a diverse group can be the difference between success and failure, growth or stagnation, life or death. A group full of warriors won't get the job done in an RPG, but a group with a warrior, a healer, a mage, a druid, and an assassin will be prepared for any situation and to conquer any foe.

I want to help you assemble a group of people you connect with on a regular basis and who are going to push you to succeed in fitness and in life. "An army of one" isn't nearly as effective as you think. Yeah, it's cool to feel like you're a lone wolf taking on the world. And sure, sometimes you are training differently than everybody else in the gym, building a business on your own terms, traveling the world while everybody else hides in their hobbit-holes, or swimming against the current instead of going with the flow.

I get it. I love being that outcast too . . . but it doesn't mean I don't also have a group of people to lean on while I'm going it alone! If you can build a diverse support system comprised of people with different levels of experience and success, you'll be far more likely to level up your life, have new experiences, and learn ways to solve problems, and more.

So let's build our group! Over the years, I've had many different groups for different aspects of my life, but in all of them I have sought a good split between character types. We might not all be the same fitness class—like warriors or monks—and we definitely are all not at the same point in our journeys either. Inspired by one of the most famous Hero's Journeys out there—Star Wars—here are the types of powerful players you need to recruit onto your team to help you complete your quests. Think of this like your own Jedi council:

* **The Jedi Master:** This person doesn't need to be some all-powerful deity you worship, just someone who has had success in the areas in which you want to be successful. If you want to get stronger and bigger and you're a skinny nerd, an ideal Jedi Master would be somebody who used to be skinny but is now bigger and stronger. If you are a single mom who wants to travel more, your Jedi Master is another single mom out there who has done what you want to do. Learning an instrument or language? Your Jedi Master can be just a year more advanced than you are, or less!

* **The Fellow Jedi:** This is the Rebel in the trenches with you, who is at the same level, struggling with the same things, and working on the same stuff. When you have a crappy day, this person knows exactly how you feel. Because you're both doing the same stuff and striving to achieve the same goals, you have somebody to bounce any ideas, triumphs, struggles, or suggestions off of in your quest toward a better life. This might be somebody who is also trying to build a business, or learn a musical instrument, or practice a new language. When you want to give up, they can help keep you accountable, and vice versa.

* **The Padawan:** The best way to get better at something is to teach it to somebody else. Think of teaching on a scale of 1 to 100, with one 1 being a complete newbie and 100 being the greatest expert in the history of the world. If you're a level 5 on a scale of 1–100, that means you can still help out people who are at level 1, level 2, level 3, and level 4. In fact, you might be better suited to teach those people than would a Level 100, because you know exactly what they're struggling with since you recently went through it! Personally, I consider myself a student first and foremost, but I have found a method and plan that can help other newbies get started with a life of adventure, which is where my business and this book come in. So, find somebody who needs help, maybe a coworker or friend who also wants to travel, or learn how to cook, or dance, or do whatever skill it is that you are currently learning. As you begin to level up, and your life starts to change, you'll begin to have people coming up to you asking how you did it and whether you could teach them. Tell them, yes.

* **The Wildcard:** He or she is the rogue/renegade in your group who is completely unpredictable: Does the name Han Solo ring a bell? The wildcard constantly pushes you out of your comfort zone, makes you try new things, and even attempt new activities. He/she will make you say "Wait, we're gonna

do what!? Okay, screw it, let's do this!" If you're not in at least one situation that scares the crap out of you while hanging out with a Wildcard, then you're not saying, "Okay, FINE!" enough. Or your wildcard isn't wild enough!

Having your own group comprised of these diverse types of Rebels will put you in the right frame of mind for advancing your training and bringing balance to the Force and purpose to your life. The people on your council can offer advice when you're confused, support you when you're down, encourage you when you need encouragement, and provide you with a constant source of motivation, inspiration, and education.

Having a support system of people I can bounce ideas, frustrations, and successes off of has pushed me to become a better person. On days when I feel like sleeping in instead of writing (on this book, for example!), on afternoons when I feel like skipping the gym, on weekends when I feel like stuffing my face with terrible food, my mind always reverts back to the lessons and words of wisdom I've learned from my "council." Even when they're not there to inspire me directly, I can always feel their presence. The Force is strong with them.

Let's dive deeper into each of these special types of players:

JEDI MASTERS

You want to pick people who have already enjoyed the type of success you're after and have shared or are willing to share their wisdom on how they did it. These can be authors of how-to books, bloggers, TV stars, your local gym trainer, a friend of yours, whoever. You don't need to personally know the people on your council; they can still be mentors to you even at a remove. Here's what you're looking for in a potential Jedi Master:

1. **They are masters of their craft.** People look to them for advice and guidance because they are truly the best of the best. Whatever skills or things you're trying to learn and build, finding people who have done it before you, in the way you hope to do it, is a great way to get started.

2. **They are honest and just.** There's a lot of crap information, false advertising, and useless products out there, especially in the fitness world (I'd guess 90 percent of fitness stuff you see on TV or read about on the Internet is effing useless or dangerous). Jedi Masters have strong convictions about speaking the truth.

3. **They are constantly vigilant, always learning, always improving.** Jedi never stop training and never stop learning. Even Jedi Grand Master Yoda continued to train, meditate, and learn new things until he died at the age of 900! You need to learn from people who never want to stop learning and improving themselves.

4. **The Force is strong with them.** Everybody learns at a different pace, has different starting points and different goals, and a Jedi Master knows how to adapt his or her mentoring approach to match the individual needs of his or her mentees. Do you need to be yelled at to work harder or do you need to be encouraged? Do you like a straightforward approach or do you need your information disguised as something else before you'll actually read it? Are you a self-starter or do you need constant sources of inspiration to stay on target?

You can find a mentor/master who can help you with whatever it is you're working on. Just figure what works for you and how you like to learn, and then seek masters who resonate with your beliefs and training styles. If you're a risk-averse, shy person, find somebody who also used to be risk-averse and shy, but who leveled up their social skills, and learn from them. Whether you want to build muscle, start a business, learn a language fast, or travel solo, I know there is a member of The Rebellion who used to be like you, but who is now a leveled-up version of themselves.

I have several Jedi Masters in my life, even some I have hired as teachers because I value their opinion so highly. For strength training and body-transformation advice, I turn to Anthony Mychal of AnthonyMychal.com. I work closely with him so I can be pushed to get stronger, bigger, faster, and fitter. After working with Anthony, I've added 100+ pounds to my deadlift, 10 pounds of muscle to my frame, and I feel invincible.

For travel and decision-making advice, I turn to Chris Guillebeau of ChrisGuillebeau.com and Derek Halpern of SocialTriggers.com. They are successful in the ways that I want to be successful, and it's fun to interact with them and have them push me to be a better boss, leader, and writer. When it comes to personal experimentation, I love learning from Tim Ferriss, author of *The 4-Hour Workweek*. And when it comes to being a great nerd and building a great community around it, I look to a personal hero, Chris Hardwick of Nerdist.com.

When it comes to building a great company that gives my team complete freedom to work wherever, whenever, I learn from Ramit Sethi, the Jedi Master who runs IWillTeachYouToBeRich.com—a must read for anybody who wants to really understand their personal finances and behavioral psychology.

If you can afford it, don't be afraid to hire a Jedi Master, too, if they come highly recommended. I gladly pay Anthony each month to train me virtually, even though I teach other people how to get fit. He's so good at what he does that I really want his specific advice on my personal situation, and I know I'm more likely to follow through with every exercise in every training session because I'm paying for it!

THE FELLOW JEDI

Sure, it's great to constantly learn from those who are older, wiser, or more advanced than you, but it's also important to surround yourself with people who are at the same level as you are. If you're an overweight single dad of two trying to get in shape, finding other dads on the same path is a great way to stay on target. Maybe you guys get together once a week to work out in somebody's garage.

Or, if you're a college-age female who wants to start adventuring, meeting up with other women at school who are also interested in travel is a great way to share ideas, struggles, and successes. On those days when we don't feel like doing the things that we know we need to, having somebody who can keep us accountable can be the difference between long-term success and consistent failure. I try to talk to my fellow Jedi as often as possible, as their positivity and success inspires me to take action and then share my successes with them. Collectively, we make each other better and keep each other on target.

I try to interact weekly with Matt from NomadicMatt.com, a fellow entrepreneur who loves to travel; Scott Dinsmore of LiveYourLegend.net (who tragically passed away while I wrote this book); Nick Reese of NickReese.com, Brian Moran of SamCart.com, and Will Hamilton of FuzzyYellowBalls.com—all friends with successful businesses. They are five of my closest online Jedi friends. We all love the idea of having a great work/life balance and helping others, and it's encouraging to talk to guys like this when I'm struggling to stay on target because they serve to remind me that I'm not alone in my concerns or worries.

THE PADAWAN

You can teach somebody something right now. Seriously. When I started Nerd Fitness years ago, I didn't consider myself a fitness expert—in fact, to this day it still says on our ABOUT page "I AM NOT A FITNESS EXPERT." However, I felt like I had an opportunity to help those who were absolute beginners to fitness, even though I was only a few years removed from that position myself.

Because I used to be a beginner, it was easy for me to anticipate beginner questions and help those who really needed it. As I helped more people, I continued my education and improved my techniques and tactics, improving my personal health and writing skills along the way. You have value, and I guarantee there is a skill right now that you possess, that probably seems second-nature to you, that somebody else would LOVE to learn about.

Along with all members of The Rebellion, my friends Saint and Helder (creator of Backlash Beer in Boston) are my top Padawan. I talk to Saint pretty much every day, offering up advice whenever he has questions on health and fitness or his own online business endeavors. We talk about app development, travel, and adventure, and it's fun for me to be the guy who gets to offer up that advice, as I was a complete newbie just a few short years ago. I have other friends I provide advice to on travel, health, business, and even relationships. I also consider The Rebellion a group of Masters, fellow Jedi, and Padawan that I get to interact with daily.

THE WILDCARD

We all have strengths and weaknesses. Although I am pretty solid in the health and fitness realm, and feel like I have a good grasp on building communities, I can also be painfully shy, a terribly picky eater, and quite risk-averse to certain types of adventures.

For those reasons, I have a few Wildcards in my life who push me out of my comfort zone. Whether it's a friend who is a social butterfly and I can tag along with, or a friend who has traveled frequently and gets me to begrudgingly say yes to an adventure (that I always end up having fun on), the Wildcard helps me grow in ways I want to grow, but that I struggle to grow in myself.

I encourage you to find a Wildcard in your life. No, I don't mean somebody who's gonna convince you to start snorting Drano or rob a bank in a Speedo, but rather somebody really great at things that scare the daylights out of you and who will help you overcome those fears.

My friend Cash is without question my go-to Wildcard. He and I have been close friends since we were in Cub Scouts together. One night while sitting at a bar, Cash half-jokingly asked if I wanted to take a trip to Peru with him, and I quickly consented before I could think twice and say no. Three weeks later I was down in Peru having the time of my life—it was an incredible experience I'll never forget, and it gave me the confidence to travel around the world by myself. Later, Cash met up with me for an adventure in Cambodia (where he got me to eat crocodile!), for trips to Germany during Oktoberfest, and to Brazil for Carnival, and it was his last-second email that convinced me to go spend three weeks in South Africa, where we narrowly avoided being attacked by baboons. I got a chance to give the best-man speech at his wedding, where immediately following the ceremony he and his bride (who had never been camping before) hopped on a plane to go climb Mount Kilimanjaro! They had a blast and will have that story for the rest of their lives. Talk about a Wildcard!

As we're progressing along our journey and completing our missions, it's this Jedi council that can be the difference between making progress or stagnating. It's this fellowship of friends that can help drive a plot (and thus the action) forward. But choose your group wisely! It's tough to change friends, and it's even tougher to admit when a friendship has run its course, but it can be an important part of growth, too. Friends come and go and, when you change, oftentimes the things you have in common are no longer in alignment, especially if those things are of a time-wasting or unhealthy nature. We have a finite amount of time—the most valuable resource on this planet—and you have 100 percent control over how that time gets spent. Surround yourself with people who want you to be better, and you will see yourself start to level up faster than ever before.

You can still have unhealthy friends and family members—I have plenty of them myself and enjoy spending time with them. Just make sure you are ALSO spending time with people who are healthier and stronger and more adventurous than you, even if it's just with friends on the Internet. Those are the people who will help you become your best self.

MASTERING ORDEALS— ACTIVATE BEAST MODE

17

PREPARE YOUR MIND TO HANDLE FEAR LIKE BRUCE WAYNE

WHY DO WE FALL, BRUCE? SO WE CAN LEARN TO PICK OURSELVES UP. —THOMAS WAYNE, BATMAN BEGINS

The next four chapters combine to form the most intense and in-depth section of *Level Up Your Life*. If you are truly interested in becoming a master of your particular craft, be it physical or mental, the next two chapters can help get you there. If you are interested in getting started with travel and adventure, the chapter on Indiana Jones will give you the strategies to make it happen. However, becoming an elite player in the Game of Life won't be easy, and you might need to make some difficult decisions along the way; that's where the chapter on Katniss Everdeen comes in. These are chapters you can come back to again and again depending on the task you're trying to complete.

To start, we must begin with the most common thing that prevents us from making progress in our missions and quests: fear. All heroes in all games and movies must confront their innermost fears. The fear of not accomplishing the quest. The fear of disappointing others. The fear of public ridicule or shame. Fear is constant and unavoidable. And that's completely normal. As the late, legendary boxing trainer Cus D'Amato said: "The hero and the coward both feel the same thing: fear; it's what they do with that fear that separates them."

I don't believe there's a better example in nerd culture of facing one's fears and using them to improve your life than the story of Bruce Wayne and Batman, and specifically what Christopher Nolan did with the franchise. Remember the scene in which a young Bruce fell down a well? He encountered a swarm of bats that would haunt him for a good portion of his young life. Eventually, Bruce decides to remove the power the bats had over him and instead channeled that fear to strike terror in the hearts of his enemies. By choosing to confront one of his greatest fears—bats—he was able to create a symbol for the protector of Gotham. If you're going to reach epic status, you'll need to confront your fears, too.

This is how the untested version of Bruce Wayne was transformed into the tough version—through identifying his fear and learning to deal with them. Bruce decided to leave all his luxury comforts behind and immersed himself in a difficult life because he knew it was the only way growth would happen. Then, through the tutelage he received in the mountains at the hand of Ra's al Ghul and his clan, his mental fortitude became ironclad.

When he later encountered another a swarm of bats as an adult, he didn't cower in fear, but rather chose to redirect that fear into becoming Batman. Those experiences forged Bruce Wayne into the Dark Knight, and your experiences in how you choose to deal with your fear will forge you into the superhero version of yourself.

CONQUERING FEAR

If we are truly interested in improving, growing, and learning throughout our lives, we need to consistently put ourselves in increasingly challenging or uncomfortable positions that scare us.

Want to know the best way to challenge yourself both physically and mentally? Do the very things that scare you! Fear and anxiety have the power to paralyze us, but they also give us a chance to acknowledge them without submitting to them. If you've ever been in a situation in which you watched somebody else do something that you wanted to do but chickened out and spent the rest of the day saying, "I should have done that," then you know what kind of power fear wields.

Let's break down the process that will help you accept your fear and then start doing things that scare you—like Bruce Wayne did in the mountains, which began the journey toward his destiny as Batman.

DECONSTRUCT THE FEAR

As I learned from author Tim Ferriss, whenever you identify something that you need or want to do but are afraid to do it, ask yourself: "What's the worst that can happen?" We often blow things completely out of proportion when we are tasked with making a decision. Getting rejected by somebody can feel like the end of the world, except that five minutes later you realize that you are now officially in the exact same position you would have been in if you hadn't talked to them—except you now get to move on instead of spending the rest of your day worrying about "what if," which is the worst!

Quitting your job and potentially failing at a business venture could seem devastating (and everybody around you will tell you so), until you realize that you've always been okay and you will always BE okay. You can downsize your house, live with a friend, sell some stuff, and get by until you get back on your feet.

If you're afraid of leaving the Shire and exploring, remember that you can always return home. Isn't that preferable to always wondering what might have happened had you gone? Heck, the subtitle of *The Hobbit* is *There and Back Again*, which is much more exciting than *The Hobbit: Not Much Happened*.

Just as Bruce had to understand that bats weren't out to get him, I want you to pick something you are afraid of, big or small, and deconstruct the fear. Whatever it is you are afraid of, take five minutes and write down specifically what's the worst possible outcome if things go poorly, and then write down what you can do to fix things if that worst-case scenario actually materialized. Short of death or a catastrophic injury, NOTHING is permanent (we haven't quite figured out the resurrecting spell . . . yet), and more often than not, the worst case is often something temporary, while the best case can be life-changing. Why surrender a life-changing moment out of fear of a potential temporary setback?

> WHATEVER IT IS YOU ARE AFRAID OF, TAKE FIVE MINUTES AND WRITE DOWN SPECIFICALLY WHAT'S THE WORST POSSIBLE OUTCOME IF THINGS GO POORLY, AND THEN WRITE DOWN WHAT YOU CAN DO TO FIX THINGS IF THAT WORST-CASE SCENARIO ACTUALLY MATERIALIZED.

If you're going to make change, and fear of the unknown is keeping you prisoner, then you need to remove the power that fear has over you. Let's say you're afraid of being rejected—what if you actually sought out rejection? Entrepreneur Jia Jiang was afraid of rejection, so he set out on a quest of 100 days of rejection to get over it (often referred to as "rejection therapy"), each day asking more and more ridiculous requests of strangers. The results? More often than not, the strangers said yes! And if they said no, he quickly learned that his life wasn't over and he could move onto the next challenge. From asking a cop to ride in his cruiser to knocking on a stranger's door and asking if he can play soccer in the backyard, Jia found himself in some hilariously uncomfortable situations. His story at FearBuster.com is worth checking out for the videos alone!

Your turn: answer the question, "What's the worst that can happen?" Most anything can be fixed, most issues are only temporary, and pretty much any problem can be solved eventually. You can get a new job, you can live with friends, you can borrow from others, you can hustle people at chess in the park. There's always a way out. Always.

However, even putting a face on this fear might not be enough to get you to take the plunge, and thus we must channel an unlikely hero: Bob.

TAKE BABY STEPS

Remember the movie *What About Bob?* In it, Bill Murray's character is so paralyzed by anxiety that he has to remind himself to take baby steps to ever get anything done. You need to do the same thing, only to a lesser extreme.

If you have stage fright, then getting up in front of a few thousand strangers might cause you to need a change of pants. So, why not start by practicing in front of a mirror. Then try talking to a few coworkers. Then practice in front of some family members, then on a street corner, then in a room of 50, and so on. Baby steps!

Let's say you have "approach anxiety," which makes you struggle with being able to talk to somebody you're interested in (this particular fear paralyzed me for years). I'm sure most nerds can relate. Rather than just going all in, which I could never quite convince myself to do, I got practice first by talking to somebody I knew I had no interest in! An elderly man or woman waiting in line for coffee, a married couple, the waiter, whoever. Because there's no chance for rejection in these interactions, there's nothing at stake and nothing to fear. You're just talking. And if for whatever reason they don't want to talk back, who cares? You were just being friendly. Once you get comfortable doing this, then you can push yourself further outside of that comfort zone until you realize that approaching somebody you're interested in could result in the same thing: a great conversation, a poor conversation (and then you know what to work on), or refusal (maybe they're in a bad mood or not that fun to talk to). There's only one way to find out!

I love to play music, and I try to play every single day, but I have very little confidence in myself performing in front of anybody: it scares the crap out of me! So I've been taking voice lessons, which has given me confidence to sing in front of my teacher. Then I started singing in front of my friends when we'd sit around and jam. Then, I played to a room full of family and friends (after a few drinks). Next on the list was performing at night on a street corner, which scared the CRAP out of me. But I did it! There's even proof at LevelUpYourLife.com. Next up, try out for *The Voice* . . . kidding!

ACCEPT IT AND RELAX

Personally, I'm deathly afraid of public speaking, but I force myself to do it whenever opportunities present themselves. My best friend, Cash, asked me to be the best man at his wedding, and after I said yes I immediately started panicking about the best man speech! I feel like Eminem in *8 Mile* any time I have to give a talk in front of people, as if I might vomit before I get on stage, no matter who I need to talk to—be it my friends or on a stage in front of thousands.

To cope with that anxiety, I simply slow down my breathing, accept the fact that I'm going to get nervous, and then tell myself, "Hey, it's going to be okay." Hell, even Sir Paul McCartney gets nervous before performing. It's weird, but simply acknowledging the fear and then laughing a bit about it ("Man I'm really nervous and freaked out, HA!") can go a long way.

DON'T GIVE YOURSELF A CHANCE TO BACK OUT

If you're afraid of trying something, burn the bridge behind you so that you have no choice but to move forward. This tactic has been used multiple times throughout military conflicts to remove the word "retreat" from soldiers' minds. Or, in the words of William Wallace's friend Amish in the movie *Braveheart:* "Well, we didn't get dressed up for nothing." Might as well fight!

Have you ever gone skydiving? Although you're jumping from a much higher spot than if you were bungee jumping, I found skydiving to be way less scary. When you skydive for the first time, you are strapped to a professional who ultimately decides when to jump out of the plane—you're in the side car, so to speak, and he or she is calling the shots. Ultimately you're just along for the ride. When you bungee jump, it's up to you to jump off a freaking bridge into the unknown. As I waited my turn to jump off Kawarau Bridge in New Zealand I watched the woman in front of me, who was supposed to jump, panic and freeze for 10 minutes before asking to be taken down and unstrapped. Nothing like watching that unfold before tiptoeing up to the side of a bridge and having to tell yourself to jump!

A few years back I published an article on Nerd Fitness about "doing shit that scares you," as I was about to embark on an around-the-world trip. I was terrified, but I'd already booked the trip before I'd given myself a chance to talk myself out of it. Later that day I received an email from an employee at Google inviting me to come talk about my Epic Quest and Nerd Fitness at Google headquarters when my trip took me to San Francisco. I immediately said yes before I gave myself a chance to say no. Of course, after I said yes I freaked out and was a nervous wreck for the entire month leading up to my talk. But I did it, and I'm so thankful I did.

If you are afraid to run a race, sign up and pay for it before you can change your mind. Prepay for those 10 jujitsu classes; if you're anything like me you'd hate to waste money already spent, so you might as well just go!

STRENGTH IN NUMBERS

Because life is the ultimate MMORPG, and because you have assembled a Jedi Council of your very own to help you along your hero's journey, don't be afraid to turn to others to help you conquer your fears.

Just like I needed my more-traveled friend Cash to help me overcome my fear of travel, and Bilbo needed Gandalf to "give him a little nudge out the door" in *The Hobbit,* you don't have to face your fear alone! If you're afraid of talking to people, recruit a friend more socially advanced than you and have them walk with you or go out with you until you develop the skill and confidence to go it alone. There's no shame in having wingmen, and often they can be the difference between a successful adventure and one that never gets off the ground. Just ask Luke Skywalker about his buddy, Wedge!

Like Bruce Wayne, you can harness the power of fear as a force for growth through the embrace of insane courage. It's easier said than done, but you're not playing this Game of Life for the consolation prize. You're playing to level up to the max—to become more than you've ever been before.

CONQUERING FAILURE

Although fear comes in all shapes and sizes (or has 8 legs), for many it most often takes the shape of a fear of failure. While the sting of failure can often be harsh and upsetting in the short term, failure can also teach you more about yourself than any success you'll ever have.

Yes, properly understanding failure can potentially trigger a more positive effect than success, if you learn how to deal properly with that failure. Failure teaches you what you need to work on, where your shortcomings lie, and what paths won't work. If you are lazy or complacent, you can lie to yourself and lie to others by saying you're trying, but failure will teach you that slacking off and coasting won't lead to success. Failure teaches you exactly what went right and what went wrong and how to improve your chances for success the next time around.

Naturally, this concept also applies to video games! Think back to the last great game you played. You make your way to a new final boss of a level, and he absolutely kicks your ass. Do you whine, mope, give up, and go, "Oh man, I'm a terrible person!"? Do you throw your controller and go, "This game is stupid!"? Hell No! You hit restart, learn from your last attempt, and manage to get a little bit better. You still lose, but now you're inspired and excited by what the future holds. When, after 10, 20, 50, 100 tries, you are finally victorious, the level of satisfaction you feel is positively intoxicating.

Now, compare that feeling to beating that same boss on the first try. Because you won right away, your skills don't improve, you don't cherish the victory, and you don't appreciate the effort required to be successful. Games without challenge are a waste of time. Famed rocker and fitness enthusiast Henry Rollins says in his must-read essay, "Iron and the Soul": "200 pounds is always 200 pounds." If you fail at picking up a weight in the gym, you can work harder and eat better and eventually find success—your friends or your brain might lie to you, but the weight will never lie.

I'd be remiss if I didn't mention another kind of failure: When you give a task every ounce of your effort—everything you've got—and you still fail. I imagine this is what most Olympic athletes who don't win a gold medal feel like. It wasn't because you didn't try hard enough, or because you were lazy—it was just because you weren't good enough at that moment, and it wasn't your time.

Although the failure still stings, it's far worse looking back knowing that you could have done more. This reaction allows you to move on without regret.

While we might not have fallen down any wells like Bruce Wayne, or been besieged by winged creatures, battling and defeating our fears can have an addictive effect for us as well. When the risk of failure loses its power and we learn that a failure doesn't mean the world is ending, taking the next risk doesn't seem quite as daunting. You can try and fail and then move on like a scientist testing a hypothesis, or you might actually succeed! Either result will teach you something about the skill or quest you're chasing, and makes it much more of an experiment than a personal reflection on you as a person.

Thomas Edison famously failed at least seven hundred times before finding the correct filament to make a light bulb. If he had given up after 699 different attempts, who knows where we'd be today? Attempt. If you succeed, congratulations! If you fail, assess, analyze, and then either commit yourself to improvement or move on! Learning to fail regularly and differently each time is just like learning the pattern of a boss on a video game and trying again to beat him.

Without taking risks, there can be no innovation. Without failure, there can be no growth. And without failure, we might never get to where we need to go. I had to get cut from my high school basketball team to find my love for strength training. I had to work a crappy job in California that led me to starting a blog. These failures got me where I needed to be, exactly when I needed to be there. The sooner you can remove the power that the fear has over you, the sooner you can get back to leveling up. Be more like Bruce Wayne and attack your fears head on.

DEVELOPING MENTAL FORTITUDE

No matter what we want to do with our lives, whether it's becoming Batman, trying to get a boyfriend, or attempting to make it as a musician, the journey is going to be filled with ups and downs. We're going to struggle, we're going to screw up, and we're going to suck and get frustrated when things don't go according to plan. Fortunately, there are specific ways we can mentally and physically bounce back from these setbacks. I've already hopefully convinced you to fail more. I'm now going to give you permission to suck more. I promise this isn't as dirty as it sounds.

> WITHOUT TAKING RISKS, THERE CAN BE NO INNOVATION. WITHOUT FAILURE, THERE CAN BE NO GROWTH. AND WITHOUT FAILURE, WE MIGHT NEVER GET TO WHERE WE NEED TO GO.

Throughout our day, there's a pull from within that tells us to stick with the things we're kind of good at, or things that we can't embarrass ourselves with. I want you to do the exact opposite of that; earlier I talked about the fear of the unknown or the fear of failure. Now I want to crush another fear we might have: the fear of sucking at something!

Take a second and think of somebody who is great at what they do: be it a professional athlete, world-class musician, or prolific artist. Here's the truth: at some point in their lives, they absolutely sucked at that activity. It might have been five decades ago, but regardless of their innate abilities, they all started at Level 0. Michael Jordan wasn't born with the ability to dunk from the foul line. Louis C.K. wasn't born hilarious. Chris Hardwick wasn't always king of the nerds: these guys all sucked for a long time until they got better. It was that willingness to push through the "suck" that got them to where they are.

No matter what we're attempting to learn on our mission, we all start at "suck." The first few steps we take on a dance floor might make us feel like a drunken giraffe. The first note we play on a violin might sound like a dying cat—mine certainly did. Our first punch in a martial arts class might look like we're asking a question. And that scares us! We're so afraid of being bad at something, so ashamed of being seen sucking at something, that we often decide to pick an easier path, avoiding the challenging activity entirely! This is the wrong attitude. We spend too much time comparing our Level 0 to somebody else's Level 50; we see their highlight reel and compare it to our actual lives, which is unfair. We listen to our favorite songs and marvel at them, not taking into account all the rewrites and revisions that went into their creation. We see the Batsuit in its amazing, bullet-stopping glory but not the 50 crappy iterations the designer went through before perfecting it. We see a player execute a perfect no-look pass but fail to acknowledge the thousands of hours that player spent in the gym honing his game.

We chalk up their success to being born with talent, but that's an oversimplification. The ability to be talented at certain things might be innate for some, but it's also something that can be learned and built on. Our favorite heroes all started at 0 with their particular task, and then they worked hard at getting slightly less bad at it, then not terrible, and then just okay before eventually becoming pretty darn good. The good news about being absolutely terrible at something is that we can only get better at it, and every little victory or improvement shows us that like anything else, we WILL improve.

How far we have to go is not the point. The point is to just freaking get started and have fun, and to get a bit less sucky today than you were yesterday. No amount of reading or sitting in a classroom (i.e., underpants collecting) is going to cure us of sucking, so we might as well embrace it, start sucking immediately, and get through that period as quickly as possible.

Author Jonathan Fields was interested in building a guitar, but was so concerned with building it perfectly that he never got started:

OVER THE COURSE OF THIS YEAR, I STARTED RESEARCHING WHAT IT WOULD TAKE TO LEARN TO BUILD THEM. YOU CAN DO APPRENTICESHIPS, BUY KITS, TAKE COURSES OR READ BOOKS. I LEARN BEST BY DOING, SO

I FIGURED I'D JUMP INTO A 2-WEEK COURSE THAT LOOKED VERY COOL. THAT WAS 9-MONTHS AGO AND SOMEHOW LIFE KEEPS GETTING IN THE WAY. OR SO I THOUGHT.

SO, I ASKED BOB [TAYLOR OF TAYLOR GUITARS] WHAT HE THOUGHT I SHOULD DO.

HIS ANSWER, "GO AND MAKE A REALLY BAD GUITAR." STOP WAITING AROUND, GO BUY A KIT AND DO IT. TODAY. "THE FIRST ONE," HE SAID, "WILL BE BAD. MAYBE REALLY BAD. BUT YOU'LL LEARN MORE MAKING ONE BAD GUITAR THAN YOU WILL WAITING TO DO SOMETHING AND THEN TAKING A COURSE THAT TEACHES YOU HOW TO DO IT RIGHT. YOU'LL UNDERSTAND A LOT MORE ABOUT THE 'WHY' BEHIND GOOD AND BAD BUILDING, AND THAT'LL PUT YOU IN A RADICALLY DIFFERENT POSITION TO DO IT BETTER MOVING FORWARD."

It's the same reason why Benny Lewis of FluentIn3Months .com encourages people to speak a new language on day one. Stop reading books, he advises. Instead, learn a few phrases and then find somebody who speaks that language and start making mistakes immediately! When I started Nerd Fitness, I was a pretty awful writer (go back and read the archives. They're still there . . . and they make me shudder) but, after months of writing daily, I was markedly less terrible at it. We all need to go through those moments of just absolute awfulness to get to where we want to go.

I'm pretty sub-par at the guitar, not half bad at the piano, and a terrible singer. However, over the past few months I've leveled up in all three skills (from Level 1 to Level 1.5 or 2.0), because I was more than okay with sucking at each of them. As I mentioned earlier, I decided during the course of writing this book that I wanted to learn to play the violin. Despite playing guitar and piano for years, the violin was an absolute beast for me (To see just *how bad* I was, and how far I've come, watch the video at LevelUpYourLife.com).

These days I'm only slightly better . . . but I'm miles ahead of where I used to be, and love the challenge.

Some might ask, "Why torture yourself and your eardrums?" Because I absolutely love to play music. Nothing makes me happier than playing along with some of my favorite songs (or struggling for weeks to learn how to play those songs). My buddy, Adam Moore, comes over once a week and we have "band" practice for a few hours. Our band's name is Hunky Tinn which, thanks to an Apple autocorrect of "Honky Tonk" (and perhaps some drinking), resulted in some 2 a.m. hilarity.

Now, Adam has actual musical talent. He used to play in a real band that put out an album, and I try as hard as I can to keep up. Because I'm having so much fun not being very good, and because Adam tolerates it, I don't feel pressure to be perfect, which would keep me from playing altogether! On top of that, playing music is making me happier, more creative, and more productive during the hours when I am working.

I want you to pick something you are absolutely abysmal at and record a video of yourself trying that activity. After that, I want you to spend 5 to 10 minutes each day (whenever possible) working on that thing you suck at:

* Cooking? Make a bad meal TODAY!
* Drawing? Draw a crappy stick figure TONIGHT.
* Dancing? Dance around your apartment like an idiot IMMEDIATELY.
* Strength training? Do your first awkward push-ups RIGHT NOW.
* Playing an instrument? Warn your neighbors first, and then BE TERRIBLE.

And then work on it each day. I don't care how much you suck now, or in a month, just that you picked something challenging that you enjoy, and that you suck slightly less tomorrow than you did today. Incremental progress is the name of the game, and not being afraid of being bad. Don't worry, everybody else is way too self-conscious about himself or herself to even THINK about how goofy you might look. I promise you.

Now, I'm going to share with you a piece of wisdom that has helped thousands of members of The Rebellion to finally take action. Be it fear of failure or fear of looking foolish while learning, fear can be absolutely paralyzing. But as Harvey Dent of Gotham points out in *The Dark Knight*, "The night is darkest just before the dawn." And though that might not be true scientifically, you get the point Harvey was trying to make: When you are challenging yourself with life-changing missions, it's going to suck and be tough before you get that reward.

BEAST MODE ACTIVATED

A few years back, I was in Brazil for Carnival, and a friend brought up the concept of "20 seconds of courage." He had just recently watched the movie, *We Bought a Zoo* (which I've since watched and really enjoyed). In it, Matt Damon's character meets his wife by mustering up the strength for a mere 20 seconds of courage to go talk to her, despite being a nervous wreck in the moments before and after. Had he never taken those 20 seconds to step outside his comfort zone, he never would have met the love of his life. "You know," Damon's character said, "sometimes all you need is twenty seconds of insane courage. Just literally twenty seconds of just embarrassing bravery. And I promise you, something great will come of it."

This concept brought to mind a favorite book series from my childhood, the Redwall series by Brian Jacques. These fantastic books are epic fantasy novels, except they replace humans and orcs with mice, foxes, weasels, and badgers. The first book I ever read in the series, *Salamandastron*, featured a memorable story in which Lord Urthstripe, the badger lord of an epic mountain, is under attack. At one point in the book, when all hope seems lost, Urthstripe channels the special power of his ancestors, activates

"Bloodwrath," and goes into a super invincible, crazy badger attack mode, laying waste to all of his enemies in the process.

While I'm probably the only person on earth who would compare *We Bought a Zoo* to the Redwall series, the concepts of "20 seconds of courage" and "Bloodwrath" are not dissimilar. The concept also bears similarity to what was written about the Berserkers in ancient Norse history. Berserkers were Norse warriors who are believed to have worked themselves into rages and then fought in a nearly uncontrollable, trance-like fury, a characteristic which later gave rise to the English word *berserk*.

If you've ever played a video game, you're probably well aware that the concept of a "temporary power up" is an important part of gaming history. In *Super Mario Bros.* and *Punch-Out!!*, it's Star Power. In *Pac-Man* (and the superior *Ms. Pac-Man*), it's Power Pellets, and in *Altered Beast*, the game hero has the ability to transform temporarily into various beasts with exceptional abilities. This is referred to as "Beast Mode!" Remember "HE'S ON FIRE!" from *NBA Jam*? Boom-shaka-laka!

If Lord Urthstripe could have his Bloodwrath, Norse Warriors their Berserker mode, and Matt Damon his "20 seconds of courage," why can't we have our own Berserker/Beast Mode? Rather than using your 20 seconds of courage or Beast Mode to go into battle, why not use those 20 seconds as a limited window of time in which you're invincible and you can accomplish anything? You can be terrified before, and you can be terrified after, but during those 20 seconds in the middle you need to do what you need to do.

Your twenty seconds of courage will help you overcome real, everyday barriers. Allow me to explain:

* ✳ **Are you afraid to try something new?** No problem, be afraid. Then turn on "ON FIRE" mode. Sign up for a class in those 20 seconds and make your commitment before you have a chance to back out. All of a sudden, you're signed up and have to follow through!

✳ **Are you typically a pushover?** Do you never stand up for yourself at work? Enter Beast Mode! The next time you meet with your boss, take 20 seconds to really stand up for yourself and present YOUR opinions. Build up the courage to begin the conversation about getting that raise you deserve. Once you're in the office and the conversation has begun, you might as well keep going. You can pee your pants after the meeting is over.

✳ **See that cute girl/guy at the coffee shop?** Normally you'd say NOTHING to him/her and then go home and kick yourself for the rest of the afternoon thinking about what you should have said. Instead, give yourself 20 seconds of courage! Be scared before and scared after, but give yourself those 20 seconds to say: "Hey, I need to get back to my friend/work, but I saw you from across the room and think you're really cute. Can I buy you a cup of coffee sometime?" Or, if that's too forward, give them a drive-by compliment: "I just wanted to let you know that you have a great smile. " You'll never have to wonder "what if . . ."

See? Great things can happen when you're in Beast Mode. If you're willing to put yourself out there—if only for 20 seconds—you'll grow emotionally, physically, mentally, and socially. You'll have all the time in the world to be scared when the 20 seconds are up.

GROWTH HAPPENS AT OUR LIMITS

In *The Fellowship of the Ring*, Sam and Frodo set off to Rivendell (and eventually Mordor). Sam pauses for a brief moment at a scarecrow that's just a few miles from his home:

Sam: "This is it."

Frodo: "This is what?"

Sam: "If I take one more step, it'll be the farthest away from home I've ever been."

Those who had regularly traveled in and out of the Shire probably walked past that scarecrow a thousand times without thinking twice. But to Sam, the scarecrow represented something monumental. It signified the dividing line between the comfortable, safe world that he had known and the potentially dangerous, unknown adventure that awaited him. It represented a specific marker that he could point to and say, "This is where I went further and did something I never thought I could do." It scared him, but it also changed him. He became the man he needed to be to eventually save Middle Earth. Had he said, "Meh, no thanks," because he was scared, and had remained in the Shire, Sauron might be ruling ALL of Earth by now, not just Middle Earth!

I want you to think of where the scarecrow is in your own life right now. Is it a mountain hike that you've told yourself you would finish but haven't attempted yet? Is it traveling outside the country and testing your preconceived notions of other cultures? Is it trying to learn a new instrument, or making a new friend, or attending an event that scares you?

Safety and the "known" cause us to drift instead of taking control. They tell us to avoid discomfort, to do the bare minimum. To stay at the comfy job or in the "comfortable" relationship that has already run its course. They keep us in our hobbit-holes, and within the Shire, rather than encouraging us to step beyond the scarecrow. Growth is dependent upon what happens outside the lines—what happens beyond the scarecrow. The unknown is where progress happens, and change will never come if we don't seek it out. You need to get comfortable with being uncomfortable if you're going to grow.

So try. Push. Reach. Be afraid, but activate Beast Mode and see what happens. You might succeed, and you might fail. And failure might end up being the best thing that could happen to you.

18

TRAIN YOUR BODY FOR ANYTHING LIKE JASON BOURNE

I CAN TELL YOU THE LICENSE PLATE NUMBERS OF ALL SIX CARS OUTSIDE. I CAN TELL YOU THAT OUR WAITRESS IS LEFT-HANDED AND THE GUY SITTING UP AT THE COUNTER WEIGHS TWO HUNDRED AND FIFTEEN POUNDS AND KNOWS HOW TO HANDLE HIMSELF. I KNOW THE BEST PLACE TO LOOK FOR A GUN IS THE CAB OF THE GRAY TRUCK OUTSIDE, AND AT THIS ALTITUDE, I CAN RUN FLAT OUT FOR A HALF MILE BEFORE MY HANDS START SHAKING. NOW WHY WOULD I KNOW THAT?

—JASON BOURNE, THE BOURNE IDENTITY

A strong and healthy body will allow us to accomplish so much more in our Game of Life. Our adventure quests will be easier, our enjoyment will be higher, and our sense of satisfaction and self-worth will be greater. After all, the last thing we want is to be mentally prepared for a quest but physically unable to complete the mission. A strong body is the natural companion of a strong mind. Whom should we look to for guidance on how to train our body for optimal performance? Jason Bourne.

I watched *The Bourne Identity* for the first time years ago, and instantly fantasized about what life would be like as Bourne—a rogue agent badass with an unbelievable ability to overcome all manner of attacks and obstacles. Sure, James Bond is the man (and I've even lived a weekend like him, as you know!), but Bond has the power and pull of the British government at his service. Bourne, on the other hand, exists outside the system, hunted by the very people who trained him. Ultimately, he's a human Swiss army knife—built for anything. Along with multiple passports and the ability to speak multiple languages, Jason has built his body in such a way that he's prepared for pretty much any scenario.

That outcome is what I want for you as you push forward on leveling up in your Game of Life. If you want to become like Jason (or a female equivalent, like Natasha Romanova aka Black Widow of the Avengers), you must train like a rogue agent, too: functional movement, power, speed, and endurance. Because he's always on the run, Jason must be able to train anywhere and everywhere and be prepared for anything. By the end of this chapter, you'll have a blueprint of how to do the same. I'm going to make you antifragile.

WHAT IS ANTIFRAGILE?

What would you say if I asked, "What's the opposite of fragile?" Most would say unbreakable, strong, or sturdy. Author Nassim Taleb, however, argues that the opposite of fragile isn't strong or sturdy, but ANTIfragile. I read Taleb's book, *Antifragile: Things That Gain from Disorder,* and I absolutely fell in love with the concept. I read it in a matter of days and, now, you could say Antifragile and I are going steady. Since discovering this concept, I've worked hard to rebuild my body and my life around the idea of becoming antifragile: getting stronger and more resilient as more chaos is introduced. Here are the core concepts:

* **Fragile:** Must be handled with care—if there is a disturbance or a variation in how the object is dealt with, this object will most likely break. Keep out of harm's way to have any chance of survival.

* **Sturdy:** Doesn't need to be handled with care—you can drop it, hit it, throw it, whatever, and it doesn't change. It's well-built and remains resilient no matter how many shocks hit it. If it breaks, it's rebuilt the exact same way.

* **Antifragile:** Don't handle with care! Throw it, try to break it, drop it, bring randomness and chaos into the mix, for it becomes stronger as a result. Like the mythical Hydra: cut off one head, and two heads appear in its place. In fact, antifragile objects can become weaker if you *don't* mishandle them!

For the majority of my life, I assumed we humans fit into the "Fragile" category, never more so than when I found out a few years back that my spine was misaligned due to a genetic condition called spondylolisthesis: essentially my L4 and L5 vertebrae don't line up. I always felt like I was one step away from a broken bone, or a pulled muscle, or a ruptured tendon. In short, I felt incredibly fragile, but over time I've come to learn that humans are actually more antifragile than we think we are. Here's how:

* If we pick up something heavy, our joints, muscles, and bones rebuild themselves STRONGER than before in case we introduce more chaos. This is the backbone of strength training. Conversely, if we DON'T partake in physical activity, our muscles and bones can actually atrophy and weaken!

* If we introduce an illness into our body at a certain dose, our body builds resistance against that illness and becomes stronger against it. This is the foundation of vaccinations and immunizations.

* We learn as small children that the kettle on the stove is hot, that animals can bite, that life is challenging. We learn from

these small bits of chaos, amounts of discomfort, and failures, and are thus more prepared to survive as an adult. If we are sheltered from everything when we are children, then when real chaos hits us as adults, we are not prepared to handle it.

Because we are antifragile creatures at heart, NOT fragile, we actually NEED chaos, disruption, and failure in our lives or we will wither and die. Remember the overweight future versions of the human population in the movie *WALL-E*, humans with zero muscle mass and a complete inability to take care of themselves? They stopped challenging their antifragile bodies, started handling themselves with too much care, spent years simply taking the easy way out—and they suffered as a result. They eliminated all "discomfort" from their lives and thus became fragile in the process. We need to do the opposite. We each need to unleash our inner Jason Bourne.

Jason Bourne is the most antifragile character I've ever encountered. The more chaotic the challenge thrown in front of him (say a government is collapsing, he's trapped in a foreign country with no easy escape plan, and he's being hunted by assassins or snipers or soldiers), the more he thrives. He has built his body with this concept of antifragility in mind. Because he has been beaten up, tested, and thrown into so many situations, he has prepared his body for survival in ANY environment.

If you want to have optimum strength and stamina for your various life quests, then you must introduce the right amount of chaos to help build your body into an antifragile powerhouse. Introduce too little and your body won't need to adapt. Introduce too much and you could get sick or injured. But introduce just the right amount, and your body will be forced to adapt and recover stronger than before.

If you've spent the past three years on the couch but then go outside tomorrow and try to run a marathon, you'll probably end up with a broken foot, shin splints, plantar fasciitis, or worse. But if you spend six months running just a few yards farther every day than you did the day before, your body will actively adapt to the situation and prepares for chaos—an increased challenge.

That increased challenge could be something as simple as increasing the length of your run from one mile to two, or running up hills or on trails, or mixing in sprints. Gradually those challenges introduce additional chaos to your system and teach your body to adapt and recover faster. That's the method we need to use to produce Bourne-like results.

THE METHOD OF MAKING ONESELF ANTIFRAGILE

If we hope to prepare ourselves for the unknown, then we need to constantly introduce discomfort, challenge, and chaos to our bodies! From a physical perspective, this means we need to provide ourselves with two things:

* Enough chaos to force our body to rebuild itself stronger;
* Enough time for our body to recover after the chaos.

In order for you to have a strong body, you need to have a strong heart. Just like you can work and overload your muscles, so too can you train your heart by challenging it! Here's an example: If every day you do the same or similar exercises that require a comparable amount of exertion, your heart grows accustomed to that level of exertion and never needs to do any extra work—until that day when you're chased by an assassin or secret agents (because you are Jason Bourne), or you go whitewater rafting, or run to catch a bus, or even just deal with a super-stressful day at work. Suddenly you've introduced TOO much chaos too quickly and, BOOM, welcome to empty heart containers and the "game over" screen.

Compare that to putting your body through an antifragile routine: run faster, run slower, up hills, down hills, sprinting, walking, hiking, cycling. Pick up heavy things for many reps, or pick up REALLY heavy things once. Now your body can no longer effectively predict what's going to happen next, but it has adapted by becoming stronger and more resilient and thus more prepared to handle chaos. A 2014 study has shown that resistance exercise can reduce the incidence of coronary events and increase survival chances after myocardial infarction, and resistance training has been shown to improve heart function in stable patients with heart failure. Yup, your heart is a muscle that can become anti-fragile, too.

Strength training, sprints, and intense bodyweight exercises all help us become more antifragile—by focusing on these movements we'll be able to thrive in power-lifting competitions, at GORUCK challenges and Tough Mudders, and keep us alive during the inevitable zombie apocalypse. We can't predict the future, but we will sure as hell be prepared when it gets here.

When this method of fitness training is put into practice, an antifragile body starts to take form. You'll know when that transformation is happening to you by looking for the following cues in your Bourne quests:

* **A low body-fat percentage:** It's tough to vault over obstacles and climb buildings or evade attackers while carrying a bunch of extra weight. We want FUNCTIONAL muscle, prepared for any situation, so more muscle mass and less body fat is key.

* **Real-world functional strength:** Isolated bicep curls mean nothing when you need to launch yourself over a fence or carry an ally to safety. We'll be training in a way that maximizes efficiency and strength without taking up all our time.

* **Tight, dense muscle:** Extra bulk and size is a challenge to achieve, but we'd rather build very tight, dense muscle (male or female) that gives us the most bang for our buck. Every pound counts when we're on the run.

* **A jack of all trades attitude:** The ability to run a 5K if necessary, sprint or swim if required, but also the strength to evade capture through training with functional movements like pull-ups, dips, push-ups, squats, lunges, jumps, and so on.

THE ANTIFRAGILE TRAINING BLUEPRINT

Imagine you're Jason Bourne (listening to Moby's "Extreme Ways" can help), and you want to stay in peak physical condition at all times. Do you spend your afternoons in an air-conditioned Globo Gym doing bicep curls and sculpting your calves in between sessions on the elliptical trainer? Heck no. You need to build a workout plan that can be done anywhere, at any time that efficiently trains your body so you are prepared for any situation.

For example, although I rarely go rock climbing, I've built my body in such a way that if you sent me climbing today, or whitewater rafting tomorrow, I could do pretty darn well. If I had to run a 5K tomorrow I could do so, even though I haven't necessarily trained for it. When I traveled around the world with a backpack for a year, I never once set foot in a gym and still managed to get myself in the best shape of my life because I learned to train with antifragility in mind.

You need a workout plan that is as antifragile as you hope to become: It can be completed nearly anywhere (no gym required) and helps you build functional strength and power. Want to know the best way to do that? Progressive bodyweight strength training, and varied short-distance running. Combine those two things with a sensible nutrition strategy and you'll have yourself an antifragile body just like your favorite secret agent.

If you are interested in building a body that will allow you to accomplish anything with a decent level of proficiency, the foundation of everything you do will be strength-based. A strong adventurer is a happy and healthy adventurer who will be up for whatever.

While adventuring, you'll most likely be training in one of three locations:

1. **Your home:** Can't get to the gym or stuck at home? Get a workout done in your living room.

2. **A park:** This was my preferred method of exercise while traveling. Find a park with monkey bars or a tree branch and you have enough to complete a workout.

3. **A hotel room or the office:** Staying at a hotel with a crappy gym? Get the workout done IN your room.

If you can find a way to get a good strength-training routine done in any of those locations, you will never struggle to build some strength anywhere on the planet! On top of that, you'll be able to complete workouts that last less than 45 minutes and challenge your ENTIRE body, building functional strength and preparing you to safely tackle new challenges.

THE ANTIFRAGILE STRENGTH-TRAINING PLAN

A solid workout routine targets every muscle in your body with big functional movements that can be completed efficiently and effectively. If the following gets too sciencey for you, head on over to LevelUpYourLife.com to grab free, simple workout plans to follow along with.

A basic workout routine will have four main movements:

1. **Legs:** A good leg exercise targets every single muscle in your lower body with just one or two movements. Squats and lunges.

2. **Push:** A push movement that works your chest, shoulders, and triceps. Push-ups and handstands.

3. **Pull:** A pull movement that works your back, biceps, and forearms. Pull-ups and rows.

4. **Core:** An exercise that targets your lower back and abs to effectively strengthen your midsection. Planks and hollow body holds.

With just four movements, your entire body will become more antifragile. The key is to introduce a challenging movement for each particular part of your body, and then continue to increase the challenge every time you complete it. If you're doing exercises that only require your bodyweight (say push-ups, or pull-ups), you need to introduce chaos by either increasing the reps or increasing the difficulty of the exercise.

If you've ever seen a gymnast and said, "Holy crap, they're strong," know that gymnasts build their strength through bodyweight exercises. What's great about these exercises is that they can be made more difficult simply by changing the angle (feet on a bench for bodyweight push-ups, wide grip pull-ups, etc.) or by using only half of the body (one handed push-ups, one-legged squats, etc.) In fact, here is my playground workout, which I've used on six continents to stay in great shape while traveling:

THE ANTIFRAGILE PLAYGROUND WORKOUT

Complete the following workout by doing three total circuits. Based on your ability, pick one exercise from each category, complete one set and move on to the next exercise immediately. At the end of Exercise E, return to Exercise A and repeat the whole process two more times. Go to LevelUpYourLife.com for a video demonstration of each move.

EXERCISE A:
EXPLOSIVE LEG WORK: 10 REPS

<hr>

LEVEL ONE

ALTERNATING STEP UPS

Standing in front of a bench, step with one leg onto the bench, and then explode with the other knee up towards the sky. Step back to the ground, and switch legs. If you can't explode the other knee up yet, just come to a full standing position on the top of the bench—that's more than okay!

LEVEL TWO

BENCH JUMPS

Standing in front of a sturdy bench, squat and jump as high as possible, landing as softly as possible on the bench with a mid-foot strike, and then step down, and repeat. DO NOT JUMP DOWN off the bench—that's how people blow out their Achilles tendons. Step down. You're welcome!

EXERCISE B:
PUSH EXERCISES: 10 REPS

<hr>

LEVEL ONE

ELEVATED PUSH-UPS

Use the back of a bench to do your push-ups. Keep your abs and butt tight and your elbows at your side. If you need to do your push-ups against a wall or a fence, that's okay, too.

LEVEL TWO

LOWER INCLINE PUSH-UPS

Use the seat part of a bench for your push-ups.

LEVEL THREE

REGULAR PUSH-UPS

If you can complete 3 sets of 10, aim for 3 sets of 20. If you can do that, make them harder by putting your feet on the bench and doing decline push-ups.

EXERCISE C:
PULL EXERCISE: 10 REPS

LEVEL ONE

SWING ROWS

Grab the chains of a swing set swing, lean back, make your body tight and straight from your head to your toes, and use your back and arm muscles to pull yourself up.

LEVEL TWO

BODY ROWS

Find a bar that's low enough, the underside of a table, a set of ladder rungs, whatever! Make your body into a tight plank, and pull yourself up. Your park might even have a bar at this perfect height.

LEVEL THREE

PULL-UPS

Standing in front of a pull-up bar or monkey bar, grab the bar with palms AWAY from you (pull-up) or FACING you (chin-up). Engage your shoulders (pull your shoulder blades back and downward), keep your core tight, and pull your chest up toward the bar. If these are too tough, do NEGATIVES—jump and use the momentum to pull your chin above the bar, and then lower your body slowly.

EXERCISE D:
LEGS: 8 REPS EACH LEG

LEVEL ONE

ASSISTED LUNGES

Hold on to a sturdy support, like the back of a bench. Take a very wide lunge stance (take a big step forward with one foot and a big step backward with the other). Make sure your stance is wide enough so that when you drop down, your front knee doesn't extend beyond your toes. Drop your back knee toward the ground, and then explode back up. After doing all 8 reps, switch legs!

LEVEL TWO

LUNGES

With your hands on your hips, step out with your right leg and drop your left knee toward the ground. Make sure you step out far enough so your right knee is not extending beyond your toes. Explode back to the starting point, and repeat with the opposite leg.

EXERCISE E:
CORE: 10 REPS

LEVEL ONE

BENT LEG REVERSE CRUNCHES

Lie flat on your back with your hands at your sides and your legs bent at 90 degrees. Flex your stomach, pull your legs up, bring your knees up, and then inward toward your chest. Lower, and repeat.

LEVEL TWO

STRAIGHT LEG REVERSE CRUNCHES

Depending on your flexibility, this might be very tough, so feel free to move on to Level 3 if those are easier. Work on flexibility until you can do these. Lie flat on your back with your legs straight, engage your core, and bring your straight legs up until they are perpendicular to the ground. Lower them back down, then repeat the process.

LEVEL THREE

HANGING KNEE TUCKS

Hang from a bar and flex your abs. Use your core to pull your knees up toward your chest. Once you can do three sets of 10 easily, it's time to move on to more difficult exercises.

If you are looking for other free workout plans, go to LevelUpYourLife.com to get workout plans that will take care of you no matter the situation, like the Beginner Bodyweight Routine that you can complete in your home, or the Hotel Room Workout for when you are traveling!

If your fitness goal is to lose a few pounds and fit into your clothes better, you might think you don't need to strength train. But by putting your focus on getting stronger and faster, and then combining that with an antifragile nutrition plan, your appearance will adjust itself accordingly. As noted alpinist and trainer Mark Twight, who trained the actors for the film *300*, has said, "appearance is a consequence of fitness."

If you are making consistent improvements with your strength and speed, the way you look in the mirror will improve as a side effect. As far as side effects go, "being ridiculously good looking" is a great one.

THE ANTIFRAGILE STAMINA PLAN

If you're somebody who wants to stay active on days other than the days when you're not building strength, there are a few things you can do:

* **Walking:** I love walking everywhere, as it's a fun way to explore new locations. It's also low impact (which saves your joints) and is a good way to burn fat without overexerting yourself. Combine strength training with walking on your off days, and you'll have a perfect plan to build muscle and burn fat.

* **Interval training:** You know how we talked about putting your heart through a workout, varying the stress it has to deal with? Interval training (varying the speeds in which you run/ walk/jog/sprint) will give you a fantastic workout in just twenty minutes. If you want to learn more about interval training, check out LevelUpYourLife.com.

* **Sprinting:** Jason Bourne can get away from captors and authorities whenever necessary because he has a fantastic top speed. Just like anything, you can level up your sprints, too. Channel The Flash, and find a hill or open field on which you can test out your top speed. Pick a starting line

and ending line, build up to a top speed, and then walk back to the starting line, rest as long as you need to, and repeat the process for 15 minutes. Complete a sprint workout once or twice a week (on non-strength-training days) and you'll increase your speed (and your heart's strength!) in a quick amount of time.

* **Have fun!** The most important part of staying fit is finding an activity you enjoy and finding a way to do it as often as possible. That could be martial arts, yoga, live action role-playing, hiking, geocaching, even playing *Wii Fit* or something along those lines. If you enjoy running or biking or swimming, go for it! Whatever gets you active and moving.

THE ANTIFRAGILE NUTRITION PLAN

Believe it or not, how you eat accounts for 80 to 90 percent of the battle when it comes to building a healthy body that is prepared for any activity. This means you need to build a kickass nutrition plan. It starts by continuing the idea of antifragility. A great antifragile diet checks all the following boxes:

1. Eat real food most of the time.

2. Don't rely on meal timing or calorie counting.

3. Do the best you can.

Let's take a look at each of these rules individually:

#1 Eat Real Food: Consume foods that existed before modern society took over: aka vegetables, protein (be it from animal sources or legumes), fruit, and nuts. You've probably heard of this type of diet referred to as "the Paleo Diet" or "eat like a caveman." It's the ultimate antifragile diet, as you're eating time-tested, natural foods that have existed for millennia. Better yet, these foods can generally be found anywhere on the planet, and they keep things simple so you don't need to worry about counting calories or weighing your food. Do you think Jason Bourne keeps track of his points while evading an assassin? Doubtful!

You might be wondering what specifically you should and shouldn't eat. Let's start with the "what," and then we can cover the "how much." Cap'n Crunch, pizza, pasta, bread, candy, soda— these are all fragile processed foods that would make Jason Bourne overweight, so we should avoid them whenever possible. We want our focus to be on quality food from natural sources (this can oftentimes be easier in foreign countries than it is in the United States, as it seems this country is built around grains, high-fructose corn syrup, sugar, and carbs!).

If you're going full-Bourne, here's what you should be building your diet around:

* **Meat:** Grass-fed beef whenever possible.
* **Fowl:** Chicken, turkey, duck, hen—things with wings.
* **Fish:** This includes shrimp, lobster, crab, mussels, clams, and other water-dwelling creatures.
* **Eggs:** Preferably Omega-3 enriched eggs.
* **Vegetables:** Dark leafy green veggies are a favorite. No, corn is not a vegetable!
* **Oils:** Olive oil, coconut oil, avocado oil—think natural.
* **Fruits:** A good source of carbs, but they can contain lots of natural sugar and can be higher in calories, so limit if you're trying to lose weight.
* **Nuts:** Loaded with healthy fats but high in calories, they're good for a snack, but don't eat bags and bags of them.
* **Tubers:** Sweet potatoes and yams. Higher in calories and carbs, but good right after a workout to replenish your glycogen levels.

#2: Don't rely on calorie counting or meal timing: Do you think Jason Bourne busted out a food scale or calorie counter to make sure he didn't go over his point allotment for the day while evading capture? Do you think he perfectly calculated his macro-nutrients on the run? Hell no!

Instead of calculating caloric intake, we're going to keep things stupidly simple. Every meal should have a protein source; every meal should have at least one vegetable; and every meal should contain healthy fats, not more carbs. When I'm aiming to lose weight or drop body fat, I keep my carb count under 100 grams per day, which is easy when my diet is built around vegetables, pro-tein, and healthy fats. This strategy will hold up in any country around the globe.

Next, I want to talk about meal timing. Do you think Bourne brought six perfectly portioned Tupperware containers with him every day in his bug-out bag so he could eat small meals scattered throughout the day? Highly doubtful. Jason was no stranger to the concept of "feast or famine," as he often would go an entire day without eating before coming to his next meal, as that's his only option for surviving!

He couldn't perfectly time his meals, and he often ate a lot or not at all. Even though conventional wisdom will tell you other-wise, recent PubMed studies and even the *New York Times* have concluded that the "eat six small meals to stoke the metabolic fire and lose weight" diet and "you must eat breakfast for weight loss" argument doesn't hold water when properly tested. In fact, this idea of occasionally skipping meals has scientific backing when it comes to helping regulate healthy weight, strength training, and more.

This is referred to as intermittent fasting: a pattern of eating whereby you feast and fast, perhaps only eating between the hours of noon and 8 p.m. and fasting the rest of the day, or doing an occasional 24-hour fast once a week. When following an eating pattern like one of these recommended two, studies have shown that fasting can lead to improved insulin sensitivity, a decrease in insulin production, and an increase of growth hormone secre-tion. In non-science terms: Intermittent fasting can help teach your body to use the food it consumes more efficiently. For many

CONTINUED ON PAGE 200

REBEL HERO

★ ★ ★ ★ ★ ★

NAME: Syreeta Gross   AGE: 36

HOMETOWN: Aberdeen, MD

After my third child, I was a sloth! I was athletic when I was younger but I got an office job and literally didn't work out for seven years. I had my last baby and was close to 200 pounds AFTER she was born. I hated my job, I ate and drank too much, I had no energy for my children, my blood pressure was creeping up, and I was too young to be so achy. I needed to do something about it and I didn't want to run on a stupid treadmill for hours so I decided on strength training.

I love sci-fi and I LOVE badass female leads and I wanted to be badass, especially if a zombie apocalypse started. One night I told my husband, "I'm going to be a bodybuilder." He just said okay, supportive but unenthused. In his defense, I'm extremely good at making big declarations but my follow-through was sketchy at best!

I knew nothing about strength training and weight rooms terrified me, but I really wanted to figure it out on my own. To learn how to play "How to Become a Badass," I first went to the library and checked out some books about the subject. I like to research, and I like to create challenges to keep myself focused. I was never able to do a pull-up even as a skinny elementary school kid, so I started researching and came across Nerd Fitness. It took about six months to get strong enough to do a pull-up but I did it! Currently, my PR is 10 but I consistently can do seven. Goal reached!

SPOTLIGHT

DAY JOB: *Environmental Consultant*

ALTER EGO: *Grossmom*   **CLASS:** *Warrior*

After my daughter was born, I also set a goal to reach 155 pounds. At the time, I was 194 pounds and wore size 14 pants. I kept yo-yoing because I didn't have a consistent schedule. The leveling-up strategy helped me break down my big goals into reachable mini-goals.

To refocus on my original bodybuilding goal, I joined a twelve week transformation challenge. In twelve weeks I lost 24 pounds, went from a size 10 to a size 4 and reached my weight goal of 155 pounds. The Rebellion has kept me motivated with content I could relate to. Lastly, as part of my overall transformation, I was able to start my own company and win the contract for a job that I love and I think makes a positive difference in the work. I train with my kids and hopefully I set a good example of how to work toward goals. They don't know it yet but they're running on Thanksgiving with me this year!

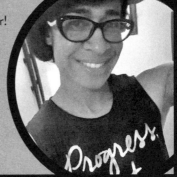

different physiological reasons, fasting can help promote weight loss and muscle building when done properly. If you are interested in learning more, check out LevelUpYourLife.com for more information and studies backing the research. Please note that intermittent fasting can affect women differently than men, so consult with your physician before making any drastic changes to your nutrition.

Personally, I've been eating like this for the past two years—I only eat meals between noon and 8 p.m. every day and occasionally follow a 24-hour fast. I've been able to reduce my body-fat percentage and increase my strength gains and build muscle while training in a fasted state.

I realize this is probably a drastically different approach than what you're used to if you've ever tried to lose weight. Many popular weight-loss plans advise you to run dutifully on the treadmill every day, eat small meals, avoid fat, and eat plenty of heart-healthy whole grains.

But do those plans really work for you? Did you get a clean bill of health? Are you able to complete the activities you want to complete and look at your body in the mirror with self confidence? If not, and if you're tired of fad diets, question conventional wisdom: try taking a more Bourne/antifragile approach to it. The Rebellion is a community of a few hundred thousand people getting results by attacking the problem this way! Try to cut out grains, sugar, and processed foods. Don't worry about meal timing—heck, skip a meal here and there . . . Put your focus on strength training, and don't be afraid to do activities that make you happy.

If any of the above resonates with you, I have a mission for you—in the spirit of leveling up your life: I want you to pick one small change to make to your diet, and do so today. Swap out fries for a vegetable at dinner, or choose unsweetened tea instead of a Coke. Do 10 push-ups or go for a 10-minute walk. But do something, and get started. After all, you need to have your body prepped and ready for anything if you're going to start going on adventures!

NURTURE YOUR ADVENTUROUS SPIRIT LIKE INDIANA JONES

MARION: *YOU'RE NOT THE MAN I KNEW TEN YEARS AGO.*
INDIANA: *IT'S NOT THE YEARS, HONEY, IT'S THE MILEAGE.*
—RAIDERS OF THE LOST ARK

From the first time I watched *Raiders of the Lost Ark,* I was hooked on the magnetic persona of Indiana Jones. Humble archaeology professor by day, daring treasure hunter and explorer by night, Indy was the guy all of us kids wanted to be. Whether it was exploring the tops of mountains, haunted ruins, mysterious caves, or anyplace in between, Indy was up for the challenge and generally came out of the experience with one hell of a story.

Okay, so maybe he also got attacked by Nazis and shot at by thieves and grave robbers, but that's beside the point. I firmly believe it's in our DNA to want to explore and to go on adventures. It's why games like *Tomb Raider, Uncharted,* and *Assassin's Creed* have done so well and spawned numerous sequels; we love the idea of wondering "What's over there?" and "What's under that?" It's the reason why those of us who grew up with *The Goonies* always hoped we could find pirate treasure in our own backyard!

In 2010, I enjoyed three inexpensive weeks of amazing adventure in Peru. It was my first-ever international trip, and I'll be telling my grandkids about it someday. The trip both inspired me and showed me there's a whole world out there to be seen. It kickstarted my globetrotting Epic Quest, and gave me the confidence to get myself into and out of any situation.

While in Peru, I went sandboarding in Huacachina, stayed in an desert oasis, hiked to the bottom of the deepest canyon in the world, rode a bike through ancient ruins and down a mountain, and eventually explored the ancient Inca city of Machu Picchu. The trip was pretty darn cheap, too. I borrowed a friend's backpack, used airline miles to fly, stayed in hostels for less than $10 a night, ate at local restaurants, and saved my money for the big experiences.

My whole experience in Peru reminded me how amazing life can be once we step out of our hobbit-holes, push ourselves to go places we've never been, meet people we've never encountered, and give ourselves experiences we never imagined. In order for us to do that, we need to channel our inner adventurer and go see what's out there.

GREAT HEROES HAVE ADVENTUROUS SPIRITS

How you've chosen to design your Game of Life is up to you. The leveling-up structure you're building and the quest lists you're making are unique to your interests and passions, and if they're not they should be. Regardless of those deeply personal choices, you'd do well to align them to your innermost adventurous spirit.

A hero's adventurous spirit is his or her engine for accomplishment—for leveling up in the face of obstacles and returning home triumphant in his or her quest. A hero's spirit for discovery in the absence of certainty, experimentation in the pursuit of learned knowledge, experiences that etch moments upon his or her soul for a lifetime—this force lights the hero's way and guides his or her decision-making when the road ahead is dark and difficult. It's no wonder, then, that the best heroes—the ones with the most awesome achievements and largest legacies—are the very same ones who truly embrace that adventurous spirit.

You need to unlock the full force of your adventurous spirit if you truly desire to level up to Level 50 status, and that can only happen if you get out of the way and let it happen. Remember, we're activating Beast Mode to get you to the upper echelon of your leveling system. I have no doubt in my mind that you, too, have a strong spirit for adventure waiting to be unleashed. That adventure may take the form of epic global travel or simple backyard adventures. The type of adventure isn't important. What matters is that you actively work to nurture this adventurous spirit as you engage in your Game of Life, one quest at a time, so that it builds up into an unstoppable force of passion and curiosity that can do nothing but fuel your growth. Ask anybody who travels frequently for adventure when they'll stop doing so. Their answer is almost always something like, "Hopefully, never. The more I travel the more I want to travel. The more I see and experience the more things I know I need to see and experience."

NURTURE YOUR ADVENTUROUS SPIRIT INDY-STYLE

Depending on the type of game you're building, "adventure" will mean different things, and your leveling system will differ from that of the adventurous Rebel next to you. That's totally fine. What's important is that you understand that adventure is out there. You just need to make it a priority and get started with the planning now! Although Indiana Jones sometimes ends up taking spontaneous trips, more often than not his travels are a result of months of careful planning, reading through old documents and journals, and setting himself up to win.

Whenever I explain to people what I've done or where I've gone, I occasionally get responses like: "Must be nice to be young, not have any kids or responsibilities, and be so freakin' lucky." But I don't see it that way. Some people see what others have done and think up any excuse or reason why they can't do the same thing.

Sorry, I can't travel, I have children.

Sorry, I can't travel, I don't have somebody to travel with.

Sorry, I can't travel, I can't afford it.

Sorry, I can't travel. I'm too old.

Sorry, I can't travel. I hear it's dangerous to travel solo as a female.

I know hundreds of people in The Rebellion who are in similar situations as those above and have still made travel and adventure a priority in their lives. I'm also going to tell you that luck has absolutely nothing to do with it. I do feel fortunate that I was born into a stable household, went to a good public high school, and attended a great university. But you're reading this book, and I'm guessing you have access to the Internet, too. This book and the Internet are really the only two things you need to start living an adventurous life today. Well, there's one more thing: A positive outlook.

Some people hear a story about somebody who's doing something awesome—like having the adventure of a lifetime, going on a great trip, or taking time off to do something fun with their family/friends/loved ones—and the first emotion that pops into their head is ENVY. "Why does he get to do that, when I can't?" they say; or "Must be nice to be able to do that. I can't because of X, Y, or Z." These people are content to sip on Haterade and tell themselves, "I can't do that, so screw them."

But those who DO seek adventure? Who DO strive to learn and grow through new experiences? They hear the same story and they feel inspired. "Hey, if he can do it, so can I!" they'll say. "Sure, I might have kids and debt to pay down, but that adventure is awesome and I want to do it, too. It might take me a few years, but I can get there."

I challenge you to remove anger, jealousy, and envy from your mind. They're not useful emotions, and they certainly won't help you level up. As I've shared throughout the book, I've heard from Rebels with families who have gone on round-the-world trips, single moms who have summited mountains with their kids, retired couples who have moved to foreign countries, and young twenty-somethings finally stepping outside their comfort zones and start leveling up. Emily Hanks is a Rebel and animal trainer who used 20 seconds of courage to book a trip to China and is still traveling. Kirsta Reid became Kirsta Sandiego, embracing her childhood love of Carmen Sandiego and now travels all over the globe teaching English! I've also heard plenty of amazingly adventurous stories from people with normal desk jobs, kids, mortgages, and weekly softball games, who have prioritized a big trip or adventure even while living a regular 9–5 life.

You don't need to quit your job and travel the world like I did (unless you decide that's what you want to do), as that was the Hero's Journey I prioritized for myself to make up for 26 years of escaping reality. However, I DO want you to start believing you have the time and resources to cross those big adventures off your quest list, and it begins with an adjustment of priorities and narrowing of goals. Below, you'll see the exact steps I follow any time I decide to plan my next trip.

PICK YOUR ARTIFACT

Indiana Jones was tasked with finding the lost Ark of the Covenant; he sought the Sankara Stones and then spent his time, energy, and effort on finding the Holy Grail (The fourth movie never happened, okay?). Every decision he made in each movie was dictated by those tasks: where to go, how to get there, what to do once he arrived, and how to accomplish his quest.

I spent years saying, "I've always wanted to travel," but never really planned out where, or what, or when. That's the reason I'd never ventured outside North America—there were always so many places to go and things to do that I never actually picked one. I didn't have my "artifact" to chase. It wasn't until my friend suggested Peru and lit a fire under my ass that I finally narrowed my focus from "I always wanted to travel" to "I am going to visit Peru, and it will happen within the next two months."

So, I want you to identify your treasure—no more nebulous goals! Pick a specific quest from your adventure list that aligns with your character type and leveling structure. The quest might be one that makes you nervous, and if it does consider it a good thing. The more specific you can get, the better. The more specific you make your quest, the easier it is to take action and get started, and thus you are more likely to complete it.

SET A DEADLINE

Set a date for when you want to begin your adventure quest and mark it down on a calendar. Let your employer know, as far in advance as possible, that you'll need the time off—so the company can plan for it. If you're traveling, put down a deposit before you can talk yourself out of going. Make the quest real.

The date you pick might be three months away, six months away, one year away, five years away, or more—just pick one and work backward from there. Our whole goal here is to move the adventure from the abstract to the concrete. Don't worry about how long you're going to go for or what the cost will be yet—we'll get to that soon enough.

To help keep your eyes on the prize, set the wallpaper on your computer to a picture of the place you want to go. Just Google "high def desktop background" and whatever country or place you're going to explore. Boom! Instant daily reminder that your treasure exists and must be found.

For the past few months, I had my desktop background set to the New York City skyline. In my continued quest to become Captain America, I figured I needed to move to New York City eventually, and I'm proud to say that I just made the move in August 2015! It's important to keep our eyes on the prize, to keep our treasure at the front of our minds. If we're thinking about it every day, it provides us with an opportunity to tell ourselves: "This is now real, so I'd better start planning."

DO ENOUGH RESEARCH TO COMMIT

Once Indy started hearing stories about the Ark of the Covenant, in *Raiders of the Lost Ark,* did he run out his front door screaming "HEY, ARK! Where the hell are you?" No, but that would be pretty funny. Instead, he researched and read and found enough information to get him started on his journey. It gave him just enough information to have the confidence to book a flight halfway around the globe, but not enough information to make him an underpants collector!

Once you determine your adventure and set a deadline, you can start to get more specific as to how you plan to accomplish your goal. I always start with a simple spreadsheet or a text document and some basic searches to get the ball rolling:

* **How long will you be going for?** Three days? A week? A month? A year?
* **Do you need to fly there?** Search Kayak.com to get the cost of your flight (tips later on travel hacking).
* **Will you require lodging?** Search Expedia for hotel prices, Airbnb for apartments, or Hostelworld.com depending on your level of comfort. Couchsurfing is free.
* **Do you need a coach?** If you're learning a skill (martial arts, dancing, a new language, etc.), use Google to search for a teacher in that area. If there are no prices listed, write down the email address of somebody you can contact for more information.
* **Are you taking a safari/adventure/excursion?** Find a similar excursion online and get the rates.

Exact numbers aren't important at this juncture; I just want you to get a ballpark figure of what you should expect to pay. I've found that for most of my trips, just starting to write things down and price the trip out, it suddenly became far more real for me than when it was just a nebulous daydream floating around in my head. For example, here's an itinerary for a hypothetical two-week trip to Peru to visit Machu Picchu:

MACHU PICCHU TRIP	COST AND DATE OF TRIP	NOTES
DATE OF TRIP	11/4–11/13, 2013	CHEAPER FLIGHTS ON TUESDAY/WEDNESDAY
ROUNDTRIP FLIGHT FROM MIA-LIM-CUZ	$844.00	DIRECTLY TO CUSCO
HOTEL IN CUSCO FOR 2 NIGHTS	$80.00	CAN STAY IN HOSTEL, HOTEL, WHATEVER
4 DAY INCA TRAIL TREK VIA PERUTREKS.COM	$545.00	INCLUDES MOST MEALS, TRANSPORTATION, ETC.
VARIOUS MEALS, ENTERTAINMENT, SOUVENIRS	$200.00	OUT AT NIGHT, BREAKFAST, TRIPS TO OTHER RUINS
TRAVEL INSURANCE THROUGH WORLD NOMADS	$64.73	ONLY IF YOUR CREDIT CARD DOESN'T PROVIDE IT
SAFETY BUFFER	120% OF ABOVE TOTAL	EMERGENCIES, EXTRA JUST IN CASE
TOTAL COST NEED TO SAVE	$2,080.48	

I know a big issue for most people is determining how much their dream trip is going to cost (I bet it's less than you'd expect if you're willing to be creative!). This exercise is designed to get us thinking about how much we need to save and by when we need to have it. If the above amount seems too expensive, even though it IS the trip you'll never forget, don't worry—there are ways to do it far cheaper, and I'll cover some money-saving tactics in the next section that will help.

Start now. I want you to spend 15 minutes to set up an Excel spreadsheet or Google Doc to get your information gathered: where will you go and what do you hope to do when you get there. Is it a safari, which you might need to plan for very far ahead? Do you need to take classes to learn a particular skill? Will you require immunizations? Can you price out your flights?

Now, just as Indy's adventures often took left turns, so too might yours. I would look into flights and the first few nights of lodging, along with any big events that might require advanced purchase of tickets. Don't overplan or overanalyze—that's the fastest path to underpants collection!

LIVE LIKE A LOCAL

In his must-read book, *How to Travel the World on $50 a Day,* Matt Kepnes, the creator of the wildly popular website NomadicMatt.com, dispels the myth that travel has to break the bank. Instead, he teaches readers how they can spend time in any country for less than $50 a day (hence, the title of the book), and in many cases much less. I've used his tactics and strategies to see six continents, doing so far cheaper than many would imagine. Would you believe it was cheaper for me to travel the world than if I had stayed behind in my hobbit-hole and lived a "normal" life? Cheap hostels, group meals, and nearly free airfare can cut your costs down significantly, and so can traveling like you live in the new country instead of living an expensive tourist life.

After all, it's tough to find spontaneous adventure when you spend your vacations in an all-inclusive Sandals Resort where every decision, down to your choice of breakfast, is made for you. Sure, there's a time and place for those kinds of vacations, too, but right now we're after adventure!

So skip the fancy, pampered hotels and save your money for authentic, real-life experiences. Depending on your budget, you can check out cheap hostels that are popular among travelers, rent an apartment through Airbnb or VRBO, and stay outside the tourist district. Consider using Couchsurfing.com if you want to travel for free! Spending time with locals, renting from locals, or going to parts of town that are off the beaten path—these are great ways to save money and experience an adventure you won't find in any Lonely Planet guide.

As far as food goes, skip the expensive meals, too! Once you get outside the tourist traps in a town, you can find relatively cheap meals or eat at carts along the street. When I traveled through Peru and Ecuador, I found delicious meals that could be had for less than $5USD. In Thailand, I found the same. Things were more expensive in Europe and Australia, but in those locations I simply cooked more by finding local markets and preparing inexpensive group meals with fellow travelers. For places to eat and things to do, consult travel sites like NomadicMatt.com or LegalNomads.com run by Jodi Ettenberg, a female solo traveler.

GET OFF THE BEATEN PATH, PLAN JUST A LITTLE

Indiana Jones's spontaneous side trip in *Indiana Jones and the Temple Of Doom* had him eating chilled monkey brains and almost getting his heart ripped out of his chest, but most side trips you'll encounter while traveling are far less dangerous than that. You can plan for some adventures, but the majority of my most memorable experiences have been from the unexpected.

When I travel, I try to book my flight in, my flight out (sometimes), perhaps a night or two of lodging, and that's it! Once I arrive in the city, I start asking locals, hostel owners, and bartenders what I should be doing or places I should be going. I take a walking tour of the city and speak with other travelers about their experiences. Just expect the unexpected and you'll never be disappointed; many times you'll get to a place you thought you'd love, but it turns out you actually hate it, or vice versa!

Once when I was in New Zealand, I was planning to spend an afternoon on Waiheke Island, off the coast at Auckland. On the ferry ride over, I noticed in the island brochure the exact photo that had been my computer background for over a year! I ended up tracking down the location where that photo was taken, stayed at a hostel with travelers whose company I enjoyed, and ended up extending my stay for over a week! Had I preplanned my entire trip I never would have been able to call an audible like that. Conversely, there have been other cities I've stayed in that I couldn't wait to leave. After 24–48 hours, I adjusted my stay from a week down to two days and quickly moved on to the next location in search of more adventure.

A recent trip to Croatia was half-planned and half-unplanned. I spent a week on a boat jumping around the Dalmatian Coast with a group of friends (I'd met them years before, traveling through Australia) for an event known as "Yacht Week." Apparently, I really wanted to be like Indiana Jones: While on the boat I managed to drop my iPhone to the bottom of the Mediterranean (where it still resides), so I had to use actual maps to get me around the country when I was alone afterward. After my first day of panic of being untethered from technology, it was pretty neat to rely on people and places to guide me rather than technology. It led me to a bus and bed-and-breakfast where I could explore the ridiculously gorgeous Plitvice Lakes. I can promise you that pictures of this place hardly seem real, but they don't even do the place justice.

When you plan last-minute adventures, or spontaneously say yes when an opportunity comes along, it removes a lot of the stress that can come with travel. Missed a bus? Who cares?! Catch the next one, stay, or go post up at a bar and chat up the bartender to see where you should go next. Once you get over the fear of not being able to find a place to stay (and you will, I promise), you don't get disappointed when plans get altered—it's tough to get disappointed when there was no plan to begin with!

If there are very popular adventures that sell out well in advance (say, hiking the Inca Trail), it's best to book those types of trips as far in advance as possible. Otherwise, simply hop on a plane, find the nearest hostel, bar, coffee shop, or tourism booth, and start asking the locals, "What part of town should I stay in tonight?" Or, "What's going on this weekend that I need to check out?" Use those 20 seconds of courage and see what happens. As a socially awkward nerd, I found traveling solo to be an amazing experience that made me hop out of my comfort zone to meet new people. I still have many friends who I stay in contact with that I met years ago on the road.

CRAVE TRAVEL? START SAVING, CONSIDER HACKING

Once you have a goal location, a target date, and a rough estimate for how much the trip will cost, it's time to start saving. Simply divide the number of weeks or months by the amount of money you hope to save (plus 20 percent for emergencies), and you'll have a new weekly or monthly amount to set aside.

Saving isn't always easy but, if you commit to it, the rewards are incredible. And if, like me, you catch the travel bug, then I invite you to join me in the wonderful world of travel hacking. If you noticed in my Machu Picchu example, the flight and lodging made up a fair majority of the expenses, as is often the case when it comes to a big international adventure. If you can use the previous tips to minimize the cost of your lodging and your food, all that's left is to find a way to minimize your flight costs. Enter travel hacking.

What exactly is travel hacking? It's a concept of learning to travel using hacks and tricks to travel cheaply. The travel-hacking community is alive with spirited folks who have ambitions and values similar to ours. They crave the freedom to experience amazing new sights, the autonomy to level up skills that may best be developed from different cultural regions around the world, and the peace that comes from appreciating other cultures and histories.

Using travel-hacking techniques, I booked an around-the-world plane ticket for 140,000 American Airlines miles and $419 in taxes and fees. Not bad for 16 stops and 35,000 miles of flying! I wrote an article about how I travel hacked my way around the world and it ended up being Gizmodo's #2 how-to article of 2010.

I've been using creative mile solutions to visit foreign countries without spending much money on my plane tickets, and then staying in hostels and spending my money instead on experiences. It's certainly easier to travel hack as an American citizen, but there are other ways to travel cheaply or hack your travel, too, regardless of where you live. Mastering this skill can save you thousands upon thousands of dollars if you're willing to put the time in to learn how it works.

Let's start with the big wins: There are certain credit cards in the United States that give you massive airline mile bonuses for signing up and spending a certain amount of money in a certain amount of time. For example: you can earn 50,000 points when you spend $3,000 in 3 months after you sign up for a particular card. Outside of spending a lot of money to earn points (1 point per dollar spent), sign up bonuses are the fastest way to accrue tons of miles quickly. Sign up for a card, use that card exclusively until you hit the spending bonus, and then repeat the process with another card. Provided you pay off your cards in full each month, you can maintain a top credit score and rack up tons of miles. Because international flights can be expensive as hell (especially if you fly business or first class), using points is the most efficient way to fly long distances without breaking the bank. I check ThePointsGuy.com daily to see which cards are offering the best bonuses, and I currently have more than a million miles ready to go for my next adventure!

Now, if you don't happen to live in the United States, you can still take advantage of some other travel hacking tactics. For example, scope out TheFlightDeal.com for daily last-minute or mistakenly priced flights that often go for far cheaper than you'd expect. If you can free up your schedule to fly on random days or change locations based on a great deal, then you can visit otherwise unavailable destinations.

Make sure you check the resources at the end of this book for the rest of my advice on traveling cheaply, including links to more information on how to make sure you redeem your miles wisely!

HOW TO PACK FOR AN ADVENTURE

You might be curious about what to pack when going on adventures that require you to stay versatile, especially if it's a trip that is going to last longer than a week. If you go to LevelUpYourLife.com I share my favorite packing tips, but here are a few basic pointers and tips to get you started:

Every ounce counts: Bring less than half of what you think you need, but more money than you think. When I set out on my trip around the world, I ended up dumping a quarter of the stuff I brought with me after a month because I never used it! Here's the stuff I ended up using regularly: one button-up shirt, a bathing suit, a few pairs of ExOfficio underwear, a few lightweight T-shirts, a pair of jeans, shorts, comfortable and versatile brown shoes, a lightweight waterproof jacket, a quick-dry towel, and a small umbrella.

Go light on the tech: If you have to bring a laptop, do so. Otherwise, your mobile phone and Internet cafes should be enough to keep you out exploring. The same is true for a camera: unless you need to bring a DSLR, take photos with your phone. I never leave home without my Kindle, as I spend almost all of my free time (waiting for a bus, on a plane, etc.) reading. Lastly, don't forget a universal plug adapter so you can charge your gadgets!

Use a backpack, not a suitcase with wheels: Everything you pack should fit into a backpack, and should be able to get carried on the plane. There's nothing worse than trying to roll a bulky suitcase through a crowded terminal trying to catch a bus, train, or plane. I use a traditional Kelty hiking backpack.

Make sure you check out the resources in the back of this book for a list of my favorite travel and travel hacking resources.

THE GOONIES GUIDE TO HOMETOWN ADVENTURE

If you're saving up for a big trip that's far off on the horizon, or travel's just not in the cards for you right now, there's still plenty of adventure to be had in the meantime. All you have to do is become a Goonie.

If you were born at any point between 1970 and 1990, you've probably seen *The Goonies* a million times. In the slim chance you haven't, or you need a refresher, it's a story about when a group of misfit kids living in a sleepy Oregon town discover a treasure map in an attic and go on a crazy treasure-hunting, mob-chasing, pirate-ship-finding adventure.

As a short, skinny kid growing up in a sleepy New England town the idea of a group of underdogs finding adventure and taking control in a less-than-ideal situation sounded pretty swell to me. I just loved dreaming that around any corner could be adventure—even in my own backyard. Maybe this is why I spent so much time exploring the woods and climbing trees in and around my family's house.

Becoming a Goonie starts with having a positive mental attitude. At first the Goonies sit around feeling sorry for themselves because their neighborhood is about to be bulldozed to make way for a golf course. Not cool. Fortunately, they discover a treasure map and find out that their hometown is in fact way more awesome than they realized. Turns out their seemingly boring little town was full of history, caves, pirate ships, and mobsters. These things were right under their noses the whole time—they just didn't know it. So stop worrying about the traveling that you aren't yet able to do and instead start to focus on the adventures you can find close to home.

You're not likely to find One-Eyed Willy's treasure in your backyard, but it's amazing how much fun local stuff there is that we take for granted. I was at a wedding recently in Atlanta, where I had lived for three years. One of my friends took his fiancé to

CONTINUED ON PAGE 218

REBEL HERO

★ ★ ★ ★ ★ ★

NAME: Pip Elder   **AGE:** 34

HOMETOWN: Melbourne, Australia

Joining The Rebellion has resulted in me changing careers, shedding excess baggage (physical, literal, and bad friends), and climbing mountains. Joining The Rebellion a few years ago gave me the thing I was missing—hope. Hope that I wasn't the only one struggling, hope that there was something better out there if I just looked.

I had accepted the fact that I would always be unhappy and unappreciated in my job, that I would be overweight and constantly struggling. Nerd Fitness changed that. The philosophy of it: it doesn't matter what your starting point is—just start, resonated with me. By going through the mindset process, I began to make myself healthier.

I gave up diet soda, which showed I could do something I never thought I could. I looked around at my life and realised that the things I thought were making me happy—junk food, lazy days, etc., where holding me back. I looked at a few people around me and went, "I don't want to end up like that." I was feeling a bit better about myself, so I took a chance and applied for the top teaching course in the country. Not only did I get in, I got a supported place, meaning the fees were much less. Not only did I love the course, I received top marks. Not only did I receive top marks, I got a job at one of the top girls' schools in the country.

SPOTLIGHT

DAY JOB: *School Teacher*

ALTER EGO: *Pipsicle*   **CLASS:** *Wizard*

Through this job, not only am I teaching my favorite subject, I am involved in a huge outdoor program that has me hiking, running, horse riding, rock climbing, mountain bike riding, and skiing every week. I've camped at the summit of mountains and watched amazing sunsets and sunrises.

I could never have taken on these challenges without the confidence that being a part of the Nerd Fitness Rebellion gave me. The confidence that to level up, you have to first beat the level you are currently on! It's a challenge, but it's not a chore.

Also—it's been my dream to spend a Christmas in London and fly business class. It's a big ask since I live in Australia. I've had this dream for the last few years and spent a large amount of time planning what I would do and how I can get there. I fly out on December 15, 2016.

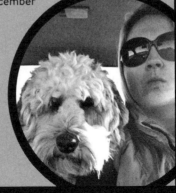

explore the city, visiting places like the Coca-Cola Museum, the Georgia Aquarium, and other places Atlanta is known for. I thought to myself, "There are probably dozens and dozens of other things I never did in Atlanta either—simply because I lived there!" It's easy to get sucked into a boring routine in your own town because everything is so familiar: you go to work, come home, eat dinner, play *Diablo III* or watch TV, go to bed.

The next afternoon or weekend day you have free, go find adventure in your city. Drive around until you find a new unexplored park or hiking trail. Go there on an early Saturday morning, bring a healthy lunch, and hike for the day! Heck, feel free to be a tourist! If you're in a city, take a bus tour. If you're in a big city, try finding a walking tour. I took one in each city I went to in Europe and they were a great way to learn about the history of the various cities. They were also great exercise. Just because it's a place you've driven past 10,000 times doesn't mean you actually know the history behind it!

Don't be afraid to use technology to your advantage, either. My favorite character in the Goonies crew is Data. This inventor of usually nonfunctional gadgets helped keep the Goonies one step ahead of the Fratellis, the evil mobsters hunting them. From flying down zip-lines through screen doors to using slick shoes to foil any pursuers, Data utilized his brain and technology to make his life better, usually.

If you're going to find adventure in your town, start by acting like Data. There's this great new fad called the "Internet" that's on the verge of taking off. From using it to find things to do in your town to plotting out a hike up the tallest mountain nearest you, there's no limit to the amount of great things you can discover in your own backyard.

How about geocaching, where you go find packages hidden by fellow adventurers? Download a geocaching application for your smartphone (or use your GPS and get the coordinates) and go on a hunt for treasure! Who knows what you'll find!

Need some ideas? Read the Wikipedia entry for your town/

city. You'll be surprised what you'll learn. Find out what they do and go do it. Consider Googling "things to do in [city], [state], [country]." I bet some travel blogger has blogged about your town and created a top-10 list of things to do there.

Now, you probably won't have caves filled with traps and mobsters chasing you to ancient pirate ships, but you can still find adventure in your backyard if you look for it. Here are some more ideas to get you started:

* **Meet the mayor of the city:** Find out who your mayor is, figure out his or her schedule, and get that photo op. Buy a comically oversized key or giant check and use it as a prop in the picture. Some day you can tell your kids you were given the key to the city. By the time you're a grandparent, you'll probably forget why you had the key in the first place and actually believe you were given it for a reason!

* **Discover "buried treasure":** If you live on a beach or near a pond, rent a metal detector and start walking. Find a watch or necklace, and you can cross "buried treasure" off the list.

* **Climb the tallest mountain:** Depending on where you live, this could be VERY easy or VERY difficult. Do you live in Florida? How about climbing to the top of the tallest building in your town?

* **Walk from one side of town to the other:** Yup. Might take you a few hours, all day, or a few days. Or, have your buddy drop you off 10 miles from your place and then find the most creative way home. Nate Damm of NateDamm.com literally walked across America, which means you can walk a few miles home.

* **Find a secret beach/hiking spot/location:** Hike through the woods and see if you can track down a cool remote spot that you can call your own. Bring a book and a lunch and have an afternoon dedicated just to you. Or bring your boyfriend/girlfriend/spouse/kids and have a great picnic.

The Goonies lived in a boring town and found adventure. I bet if you actively focus on finding adventure in your town, there's no limit to the types of things that you and your friends or family can get into. Heck, you might even find actual buried treasure or real pirates, but hopefully not real mobsters.

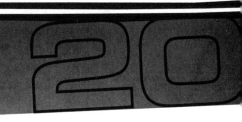

MAKE SACRIFICES THAT EMPOWER YOUR CAUSE LIKE KATNISS EVERDEEN

I VOLUNTEER! I VOLUNTEER AS TRIBUTE!
                    —KATNISS EVERDEEN, THE HUNGER GAMES

F ew moments in popular contemporary literature conjure up as much emotion as the pivotal scene in Suzanne Collins's *The Hunger Games*, in which the Capitol selects which children will fight to the death in the titular tournament. It's at this moment that we learn just what kind of hero the protagonist Katniss Everdeen will be, as she volunteers as tribute to join the tournament—almost certainly signing her own death sentence—to save the life of her sister. I remember reading those pages and my jaw dropped as I realized the gravity of Katniss's sacrifice. Yet a closer look at our favorite films and books reveals that great sacrifice is often required of the hero along his or her journey or to achieve transformation and reach his or her full Level 50 potential.

Whether it's Darth Vader at the end of *The Return of the Jedi,* Captain America at the end of *The First Avenger,* Optimus Prime in *Transformers: The Movie* (the animated 1986 version), Iron Man in the climax of *The Avengers,* or Harry Potter toward the end of his journey. Our heroes are often faced with a choice that will decide the fate of mankind and that requires them to sacrifice everything they hold dear, including, at times, their own lives.

It's these sacrifices that bring the story to the third and final act, as well as prompts the hero to arrive at the final few steps of the Hero's Journey. Without Harry Potter's sacrifice, Volde—um, "He who must not be named"—would have continued to bring terror to wizards and muggles alike. And while nobody is asking you to lay down your life here, make no mistake: if you truly want to complete your Hero's Journey, sacrifices will be required of you, too.

If you are going to become who you have decided it's your destiny to be and level up all the way up to Level 50, then you are going to face a tremendous number of choices along the way (especially as you get closer to elite status). Ultimately, we are faced with a choice every time we spend our money or choose how to spend our time, and in order for us to prioritize adventure, something else must take a back seat. To level up with other elite players, others must fade from "supporting role" to "extra." If you're going to build a body like Jason Bourne's or have the mental fortitude of Bruce Wayne, it might require you to put short-term gratification on hold and sacrifice certain comforts in order for you to grow.

I VOLUNTEERED AS TRIBUTE FOR MY FUTURE

On my own Hero's Journey, I initially refused the call to adventure. I had the idea to start my own website but, because I was spending so much time at my day job, playing video games on weeknights, partying on weekends, and traveling for a long-distance relationship, I never found the time to make it happen. This refusal of the call to step up and work on Nerd Fitness went on for well over a year, and it wasn't until my computer essentially blew up that I decided to give up playing video games until I had made my first dollar online.

At the time my initial impetus for building my own business was so I could become location-independent and spend more time with my long-distance girlfriend. The fried computer was the call to action I needed to get my act together and start on my journey to a leveled-up life. Even though all my friends begged me to spend a few hundred bucks to get my computer fixed and get back in the raids, I swore off video games. I spent far fewer nights and weekends out drinking and, instead, spent those nights furiously typing articles and connecting with readers.

I was then faced with a really difficult decision regarding my relationship, which I decided to end. I didn't know at the time if I was making the right decision, but something in my gut told me I was. It seems so obvious now, looking back, but if you've ever struggled to get out of a relationship that isn't quite right, you know it can feel like a sacrifice.

As more and more of my time got dumped into Nerd Fitness, less and less of my time was free for friends, parties, and gaming. I figured that if I could continue to delay my gratification of short-term, ephemeral desires and keep myself focused on my long-term goals, it would benefit me in the long run. I then had to make a decision about my job that resulted in nearly everybody thinking I was absolutely crazy. I had a fantastic job that allowed me to spend a majority of my time around the music industry and frequently sent me on cruise ships to the Caribbean with some of my favorite musicians. I lived with great friends, and I had a pretty damn good thing going. And then I quit.

I quit because I decided that in order for my Hero's Journey to progress—to become what I felt I had the potential to become—I would have to give up that comfortable and perfectly fine existence for the chance at something better and more fulfilling. Since then, it's been a rollercoaster ride of emotions, late nights, early mornings, and many more noes than yeses, but I wouldn't change it for the world.

Lastly, I think it's appropriate to mention that I'm currently typing this sentence at 11:50 p.m. on a Friday evening, while one group of friends is out having fun and another is playing *League of Legends*. Of course, I would love to be drinking beers with friends or playing video games, but I've prioritized the completion of my book-writing quest as part of my Hero's Journey. And as I've put a bigger focus on playing music and making fitness a priority as well, I've had to make more sacrifices with regard to how often I meet friends out for drinks or how much time I spend out late. As a result, my friendships have evolved and the game I'm playing has changed.

It's tough to let go of old friendships and old relationships. It's brutally difficult to give up on something that is "perfectly fine," especially when everybody around you is telling you that you're lucky to be in the situation you're in, be it a comfortable job or safe relationship. But if you've read up to this point, then you know that it's not about being "perfectly fine." It's about seeking adventure, completing the Hero's Journey, and never having to look back and ask, "What if?"

Because the cause behind the adventure is bigger than just you, it's now time for you to channel your inner Katniss Everdeen and volunteer as tribute so you can make a real difference, transform into your best self, and truly level up in the Game of Life.

MAKE YOUR CAUSE BIGGER THAN YOU

In *The Hunger Games*, we never would have witnessed Katniss's potential for true greatness if she hadn't volunteered to take her sister's place in the tournament. And all hokeyness aside, I know there is greatness within you, too. I actually believe this of everybody, but very few people ever truly live up to their potential. They're either unwilling or unable to make the decisions and choices required of them to level up, or they're afraid of stepping outside a comfortable but unfulfilling existence to take a risk at finding out what could be.

Imagine that the future leveled-up version of you just had its name drawn to participate in the Hunger Games, effectively sentencing you to death. Will you to choose to let your future self get sacrificed in the games, or will you instead volunteer yourself as tribute?

Before you choose, be mindful of the fact that your decision will have an impact beyond just your own "life" and "death." When we eschew the ordinary world in search of adventure down the road less traveled, we need to be thinking on a grander scale. For instance, if you decide to give up a well-paying but unfulfilling job to try something that truly challenges you (which might require selling your car or downsizing your house or opting out of the rat race), you will get more than your fair share of "Why are you throwing your life away?" comments from people in your life, even well-meaning people who love you and think they have your best interests in mind. The important thing to remember is that you're doing it to pay respect and tribute to all those people who, on their deathbeds, looked back and said: "I wish I had had the courage to live a life true to myself, not the life others expected of me."

Katniss initially volunteered as tribute as a gesture to save just her sister's life, but her decision ended up having a ripple effect with far greater consequences than she originally intended. Each day, decisions you make that seem like they're only impacting you and your happiness or life also have the potential to affect others. Deciding to skip a workout to go drinking or spend another month putting off that project to play the latest game release might not seem like a big deal, but each of these decisions adds up over time.

The truly elite players of the Game of Life understand that every decision they are faced with represents a chance to get closer to or further away from their goals. If they are seeking to reach the highest level of their game, more sacrifice will be required of them. Old friends, old habits, old eating styles, old game favorites, old relationships, old occupations—some or all of these things might need to be sacrificed to achieve this goal. So it starts with us remembering what we're fighting for, and keeping this at the front of our minds whenever we are faced with a decision to step forward or stay back. Heroes don't exist in a vacuum. Just as Katniss stepped forward as tribute to save the life of her sister, so, too, do you have the power to lift up those around you when you rise to become your best self.

In *Harry Potter and the Deathly Hallows*, when Harry finally realizes what is required of him in order to defeat the Dark Lord, he marches into the Forbidden Forest to face the Death Eaters alone. Except that he's not alone—he's surrounded by the ghosts of those who loved him, cared for him, and were impacted by his life. They give him the courage to carry on, even when all hope seems lost. Harry's scared out of his mind, but he knows what's at stake. One look at Katniss's face as she approaches the stage to volunteer tells us the same story: these are two characters who are terrified, but they are fighting for something far greater than themselves.

I want the same thing for you. I want you to understand that this is a fight much greater than simply saying no to pizza or skipping a night of drinking to work on a project that makes you feel alive: it goes much deeper than that. Are you fighting to get healthy so that you can find love and start a family of your own? Are you fighting for a better life for you and your family? Are you fighting to feel alive for the first time in years? Are you honoring your ancestors who came before you and fought so hard to give you an opportunity at freedom and happiness? Think of how the United States became a melting pot of world cultures: Immigrants went on their own Hero's Journey, traveling from countries like Ireland, China, Poland, Russia, Italy, and Germany in the 19th and early 20th century, leaving behind a normal life back home to explore and make a living on the other side of the planet. Your future self is at risk, and the world needs you to step up and volunteer your current self as tribute.

WHAT WILL YOU VOLUNTEER TO DO AS TRIBUTE?

Want to know what separates the "I'll get to it some day" people from the "already did it" heroes? The ability to say yes to the right opportunities and no to the wrong ones—the ability to actively choose to build and prioritize around adventure and to willingly sacrifice certain things that might bring immediate comfort. I hope none of us are ever faced with true life or death choices like the those faced by Katniss and Harry, but in a sense we all are. Our lives hang in the balance, because life goes far beyond the mere beating of our hearts. If we are not doing the things we love, surrounded by the people we love, and challenging ourselves to grow and make an impact on the lives of those around us, then we are doing a disservice to all those who never got the chance, or who realized their folly too late—or, more important, to those who willingly sacrificed to help make our opportunities possible.

So I ask you: What are you willing to volunteer and sacrifice to give yourself and your loved ones a chance at true happiness? If you don't mind, I've got a few suggestions:

SACRIFICE YOUR UNHEALTHY RELATIONSHIPS

It's tough to admit when the attitudes expressed by our old friends or love interests might no longer align with our new lifestyle. These are the friends who make fun of you for wanting to go bed early so you can run a race in the morning; or the boyfriend or girlfriend who constantly tells you to stop worrying about improving your health, even though it's really important to you; or even family members that tell you to shut up and be happy instead of striving for a life they think is unrealistic, dangerous, or unattainable. Sometimes, you need to fire your friends, and even fire certain family members if they're proving to be truly destructive to your interests and are uninterested in joining you on your new journey. It's painful and difficult, but these people aren't ready or willing to change or to accept change in you. That's totally fine. You can't control what you can't control, so focus on yourself and your personal development and become an example for them to aspire to. Life will go on, and you will find that there are plenty of forward-thinking people out there who will support and celebrate your new path in life. Off the top of my head, I can think of a few hundred thousand Rebels who would love to aid you in your quest!

SACRIFICE UNHEALTHY CREATURE COMFORTS

I think by now we've established that I love video games. They shaped my childhood, inspired this book, and I still play them occasionally. But by necessity they have been relegated to a back seat in my day-to-day life. It's not because I'm going away from my roots or because I have outgrown them, but simply because I only have so many hours and so much attention span to give. So I have to prioritize things—fitness or personal development or playing music—over gaming. Every few months I'll set aside a week to go absolutely nuts and play through the newest game in a series I love (God of War, Uncharted, The Legend of Zelda, Assassin's Creed, etc.), but I know myself well enough that if I were to start playing *World of Warcraft* my life could fall apart.

On top of that, in the first few years of running Nerd Fitness, everything I owned fit in a single backpack. I wore the same few outfits over and over again for years, and it wasn't until I set up a permanent home in Nashville that I finally stopped dressing like a broke college student (at the tender age of 28!). It wasn't because I couldn't afford nicer clothes. It's just that they didn't fit into my plan for leveling up until my move to Nashville. Any money that could have been spent on more gadgets or more clothes was dumped back into the business, spent on life-changing adventures, or on books and classes that would help me cross more goals off my list.

I'm not telling you to give up things you love and that bring you small amounts of joy; instead, I'm asking you to dig deep and really look at how you're spending your time and money, and decide what's really important to you. Over the past few years, I've come to learn that money spent on experiences can bring far more lasting happiness than money spent on objects. For me, I had to put gaming and many other basic creature comforts on hold for a few years so I could dedicate myself fully to building my business. While many of my friends were getting married and starting families, I put my social life on hold and instead chose to raise Nerd Fitness.

People often tell me how it "must be nice to not have a family and kids so you can travel whenever you want and not have any responsibility." To those people I would say "it must be nice to have a family that loves and supports you and children who make you feel complete! I hope I can be that lucky some day." I chose to get my life together and really learn what's important to me before focusing on that phase of my journey, but I'm confident that when the time comes I can find a way to raise a family and still prioritize adventure—as I know many members of The Rebellion who you've read about in this book already have.

SACRIFICE UNHEALTHY LIFESTYLE CHOICES

My friend Adam often jokes with me, saying things like, "I really hope all this fitness stuff is worth it. You know how good pizza and ice cream is, right?" Well, my favorite food is chicken parm, and I love New York style cheese pizza. LOVE IT. I could eat those two things every day for the rest of my life and be perfectly content. But I would also be perfectly round and struggle to live like Jason Bourne—so I take an active role in how I fuel my body. I drink less now than I did years ago, I'm in bed and up much earlier, and I have to make many more sacrifices when it comes to my choices for every meal. Although I do actively choose to eat pizza or drink beer occasionally, I know those things aren't helping me progress in my quest to become stronger and healthier, so I'm more selective in my adult beverage choices and try to minimize how frequently I drink them.

If you're overweight and unhappy and interested in adventuring, you might need to make more sacrifices when it comes to the comfort foods that provide you with temporary happiness. We are what we eat, and how we fuel our bodies will determine 80–90 percent of our success or failure in becoming healthy. The more good decisions you can make with regard to your diet, the more likely it is you'll reach that level of physical fitness required of the adventures you hope to complete. I can promise you that the yearnings for these sacrifices up front start to fade once you realize you can eat great food that's also good for you, and still occasionally eat the bad stuff without much consequence.

SACRIFICE THE HOBBIT-HOLE

This is elite-level stuff, and you'll often get tons of flack for it, but sometimes sacrificing your part in the rat race is necessary in order to grow. I had to quit my job (twice) in order to get started on my Hero's Journey. Both decisions required me to downsize my lifestyle and drastically cut my expenses. Sometimes elite-level living can only come when you are spending your day on a job that is challenging and aligned with your skills (and ideally your passions). If your current day job doesn't qualify, no amount of money or number of "be thankful you have a job in this economy" comments will change that. Your journey might require this big sacrifice if it's blocking your future. Hopefully, the job you have allows you to be who you are and gives you enough free time to do the things you want to do. Indiana Jones can be both an adventurer and archaeology professor, and plenty of members of The Rebellion work regular jobs and then live out their free time as superheroes.

However, there are definitely instances in which the sacrifice of a crappy job or a pivot to a different career path is the only choice. As the saying goes, "It's better to be on the bottom of the ladder you want to climb than at the top of the one you don't." There's no such thing as "it's too late to change." You might need to sacrifice (there's that word again) nights and weekends to take classes in a field that you hope to switch to, or you might need to sacrifice that big house and new car every two years for a small apartment to take a lower-paying job in a field you enjoy working in, but it will be worth it in the long run.

THE REBELLION NEEDS YOU

Just as Katniss's sacrifices inspired a movement, and Harry's sacrifices saved the Wizarding world, your sacrifices can help you save yourself. Not only that, but even if they don't admit it or mention it, I guarantee that when you start to live a life that's true to yourself, you'll inspire others in your life—even those who scoff and ridicule you for your sacrifices—to make better life choices themselves. Success, growth, happiness, and leveling up are all additive, addictive, and contagious behaviors. I know that my game can help inspire my friends, just as I know that my decisions are influenced by other members of the Rebellion. Beyond that, I know I have a responsibility to the community as a whole to find out what I'm capable of. I want to honor those whose sacrifices paved the way for the opportunities I've been granted in life, and I want to realize my potential. I was fortunate enough to know all four of my grandparents, three of whom have passed away since I started my journey in 2010. I'm constantly thinking of them: my Grampy, who had to help raise his brothers and sisters during the Depression and contracted malaria during World War II in the Pacific (he passed away while I was in Peru); my Grampa, who also fought in the Pacific Theater and worked hard to provide for his family (he passed away while I was in Chicago); and my Nana, who always told me "of course you can" (she passed away while I was in Cambodia). I want to honor their memory by living a life they would be proud of.

Socrates, one of the original nerds, once said (most likely in Greek): "No man has the right to be an amateur in the matter of physical training." "It is a shame for a man to grow old without seeing the beauty and strength of which his body is capable." Although I completely agree that this applies to how we treat our bodies, I think this also applies to how we treat our minds and our adventurous spirits. I honestly feel like I have a responsibility to The Rebellion and the rest of the human race to strive to reach my potential. I want to impact as many lives as I can, help as many people as I can, and I want to leave this planet a better place than when I arrived.

The Rebellion needs you to become the best version of yourself as well. If you follow the lessons you just learned from Bruce Wayne, Jason Bourne, Indiana Jones, and Katniss Everdeen, you'll be well on your way to becoming an elite player in the Game of Life. You'll be prepared for any physical challenge, ready to go on any adventure at the drop of a hat (or fedora?), and make the right decisions to advance your story.

Where that story leads is completely up to you. And that's the best part. Every quest is an opportunity to learn more, and then it's time to begin the journey home so you can start planning the next one.

SECTION 6

THE ROAD BACK— CONTINUE? OR GAME OVER?

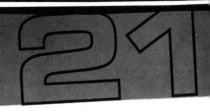

CELEBRATE THE REWARDS OF YOUR JOURNEY AS THEY'RE ACHIEVED

ALL WE HAVE TO DO IS DECIDE WHAT TO DO WITH THE TIME THAT IS GIVEN TO US.

—GANDALF THE GREY, THE FELLOWSHIP OF THE RING

Welcome to the third and final act of your Hero's Journey, my dear Rebel friend. Triumph may be fleeting, and we must begin our journey back to reality, but for now we can enjoy the victory earned after completing a trip or crossing an important item off your quest list in Game of Life. Consider this the throne-room scene in *Star Wars Episode IV: A New Hope,* or the moment when the credits roll after you've completed a video game. Yep, there's always another game to move on to, but for the time being you get a brief moment to celebrate your accomplishment and revel in the victory. As pointed out by Christopher Vogler in *The Writer's Journey*:

> WE SEEKERS LOOK AT ONE ANOTHER WITH GROWING SMILES. WE'VE WON THE RIGHT TO BE CALLED HEROES. FOR THE SAKE OF THE HOME TRIBE WE FACED DEATH, TASTED IT, AND YET LIVED. FROM THE DEPTHS OF TERROR WE SUDDENLY SHOOT UP TO VICTORY. IT'S TIME TO FILL OUR EMPTY BELLIES AND RAISE OUR VOICES AROUND THE CAMPFIRE TO SING OF OUR DEEDS. OLD WOUNDS AND GRIEVANCES ARE FORGOTTEN. THE STORY OF OUR JOURNEY IS ALREADY BEING WOVEN. YOU PULL APART FROM THE REST, STRANGELY QUIET. IN THE LEAPING SHADOWS YOU REMEMBER THOSE WHO DIDN'T MAKE IT, AND YOU NOTICE SOMETHING. YOU'RE DIFFERENT. YOU'VE CHANGED. PART OF YOU HAS DIED AND SOMETHING NEW HAS BEEN BORN. YOU AND THE WORLD WILL NEVER SEEM THE SAME.

If you're still reading this book, the likelihood is that you are alive. And that's a pretty damn good place to be. After all, the reason we play games and read books and watch movies is not so we can check off a box, but to have fun. And to remind us that being alive is amazing. Although I'm a huge fan of goal setting and completing missions—which by this point in the book should come as a surprise to nobody—research and personal experiences have shown me there also are other important factors when it comes to happiness and success. We all know that properly structured goals can give us a path to follow for life improvement. However, if we're not careful, we can spend ALL our time working on goals, doing things that help us reach the next level, but never take time to appreciate the things we just accomplished!

This is an important part of the Hero's Journey we are all on. We can't forget to enjoy the process or to remind ourselves that tomorrow isn't guaranteed. Not to be morbid, but you could get hit by a bus five minutes from now! Heck, you could discover you have a life-threatening illness, or something could go horribly wrong. We hear story after story about things like this every day, never thinking it can happen to us . . . until it does. We have a finite amount of time on this planet, just like we have a finite number of quarters to feed into an arcade game before our time is up. So we need to enjoy ourselves while we can.

As you're creating your goals and crossing them off, don't forget to think about WHY you have those specific goals, and whether crossing them off will really bring you happiness. We've all heard the stories of famous people who died far too young, whether it's Michael Jackson, Robin Williams, or Janis Joplin—people who seemingly had everything and yet struggled to find happiness. We often think the end result will produce happiness, when in fact happiness is not an end goal that we chase, but rather a consequence of the things we are chasing.

Whether it's obtaining six-pack abs, finally buying the car of our dreams, making a certain amount of money, or crossing off a big item on our quest list, our brains can quickly adjust and make this accomplished goal our new normal. Every time we complete a quest or mission, we have to remember that it's often the journey that produces the happiness, not just the destination. Put in nerd terms, it's playing the game that's fun too, not just completing it.

So, along with goals, quests, and missions there are two other crucial pieces to our happiness equation that are missing. The first is to remember that every day you wake up is a good day to be alive—it certainly beats the alternative. The second is to remember that it's not things that will make us happier, but rather the experiences we have in the pursuit of "mission complete" that produce the happiness.

I often talk about how we don't get to pick the "level of difficulty" we play on in the game of life. Some people get to play on Easy while others have to play on Legendary. While writing this book, I received the really sad news that my good friend, Tiffany Green, passed away at the age of 31 due to complications from surgery. If there's anybody who played the Game of Life to the best of her ability, it was Tiffany. In fact, she played on a level two steps above Legendary, as she'd been forced to deal with a tremendous number of medical issues ever since she was born, each more challenging than the previous. Despite all this, she never once failed to sport a smile or a positive attitude. She simply played the hand she was dealt to the best of her ability, smiling until the very end. She never complained or asked "Why?"

While doing final edits on this book, I learned that one of my good friends, Scott Dinsmore of LiveYourLegend.net, died tragically due to a rock-slide while climbing Mount Kilimanjaro. Only thirty-three years old, he died while living out his dream of traveling around the world and building a life of stories. It's a shame that it takes a tragedy to remind us how short and unpredictable life can be, and that we need to enjoy every day. The stark realization is that in order to live our lives fully and happily, we have to remember that we, unlike our video game heroes, have no extra lives. This is it. If Scott was here today, he would ask what kind of legend you're leaving behind, and how can you start living it RIGHT NOW?

I receive emails daily from people who are in crappy situations or are unhappy about the path they're on, and my advice to them is generally the same: You MUST find a way to be happy today, because tomorrow isn't guaranteed. Yes, that's easier said than done. But if you follow the techniques and tactics in this book, and you actively work on bettering yourself, making those around you better, and being grateful each day for the opportunity you've been given, you truly can level up your life. Here's how:

BE PRESENT

The Legend of Zelda: Ocarina of Time is a fantastic example of a structured game that also encourages fun for fun's sake. Although it had a clear, logical progression from one dungeon to the next, from one level to the next, there was also something you could spend hours doing purely for fun: fishing! I once took an entire afternoon to just hang out at the fishing pond. There was no score being kept, no level to complete, no quest to master. Just a leisurely activity to eat up a few hours and have some fun.

There have been some other incredible games that have come out recently that don't keep score at all; instead, they allow you to zone out and just enjoy the experience. Games like *Flower* and *flOw* are more of an experience and an art form than games in the traditional sense. The same is true for the PS3 game *Journey*. Sure, the point is to get to the top of the mountain, but it's the journey itself that brings you the satisfaction, not just the final climb to the peak.

If you are climbing a metaphorical mountain, or a real one, take a moment on the hike to relish the journey and the view before climbing down and moving on to the next mountain. My challenge to you today is to take a few minutes performing an activity that helps you be present and stop looking ahead to the future. We can find this in exercise, our work, our hobbies, and spending time with our friends and loved ones. If you want more specifics, think of those moments in your life when you've looked at the clock and said, "How the hell did it get so late?" When we lose track of time, we can't help but smile.

For me, it's playing music and attending concerts. That's why I make sure to play music every day, alone or with friends. There's something meditative about music for me that allows me to get lost in it. Music offers me a chance to shut off my overactive brain and just focus on the keys of the keyboard or my fingers on the fret of a guitar. Singing along to a song by Gaelic Storm is a chance to remember: "Here's to one more day above the roses."

For you, it might be playing video games, visiting with

> EVERY TIME WE COMPLETE A QUEST OR MISSION, WE HAVE TO REMEMBER THAT IT'S OFTEN THE JOURNEY THAT PRODUCES THE HAPPINESS, NOT THE DESTINATION.

friends, sharing a quiet beer at a pub with a significant other, volunteering, reading a book in the park, hiking alone with your thoughts, sitting under a tree with a guitar, dancing, practicing martial arts, painting, drawing, or whatever brings you joy. Hell, maybe you just want to do NOTHING—that's okay, too. I don't care your level of skill in whatever activity you choose—if you are enjoying it and it reminds you that you are above the ground for at least one more day, find a way to complete that activity every day.

If you've seen *The Shining*, remember: "All work and no play makes Jack a Dull Boy." Or, as author Daniel Pink points out in his book, *Drive*, all work and no play can ruin your day. He cites a study in which people were instructed to "act in a normal way, doing all the normal things you have to do, but not doing anything that is 'play' or 'non-instrumental'":

> PEOPLE WHO LIKED ASPECTS OF THEIR WORK HAD TO AVOID SITUATIONS THAT MIGHT TRIGGER ENJOYMENT. PEOPLE WHO RELISHED DEMANDING PHYSICAL EXERCISE HAD TO REMAIN SEDENTARY. ONE WOMAN ENJOYED WASHING DISHES BECAUSE IT GAVE HER SOMETHING CONSTRUCTIVE TO DO, ALONG WITH TIME TO FANTASIZE FREE OF GUILT, BUT COULD WASH DISHES ONLY WHEN ABSOLUTELY NECESSARY.
>
> THE RESULTS WERE ALMOST IMMEDIATE. PARTICIPANTS "NOTICED AN INCREASED SLUGGISHNESS ABOUT THEIR BEHAVIOR." THEY BEGAN COMPLAINING OF HEADACHES. MOST REPORTED DIFFICULTY CONCENTRATING. SOME FELT SLEEPY, WHILE OTHERS WERE TOO AGITATED TO SLEEP. THE DETERIORATION IN MOOD WAS SO ADVANCED THAT PROLONGING THE EXPERIMENT WOULD HAVE BEEN UNADVISABLE. ALL OF THIS HAPPENED WITHIN 48 HOURS.

Here is actual evidence that not spending time on things we enjoy each day can put us on the fast track to a miserable existence. It is therefore essential we carve out time daily for the things we truly enjoy, even if it's just a few minutes. If you spend all your time working and stressing yourself out, you can get burned-out pretty easily. Even worse, you can grind for decades before realizing that you've spent your life like a countdown clock: counting down to the weekend, counting down to summer vacation, counting down to the end of the work day. If you're currently living every day like a countdown clock, it might be time to mix things up. Steve Jobs once said: "I have looked in the mirror every morning and asked myself: 'If today were the last day of my life, would I want to do what I am about to do today?' And whenever the answer has been 'No' for too many days in a row, I know I need to change something."

It's amazing how much happier you can be when you realize you have the opportunity and ability to enjoy the life that you are CURRENTLY living. Yesterday already happened. You can't control tomorrow. So why not focus on being happy today?

BE GRATEFUL

There's one final life hack I want to share with you that will lead to you being happier every single day: Practice gratitude. Oftentimes the source of our unhappiness is because we spend our time wishing we were like somebody else, or that we had something else, or that we were doing something else. If our reality exceeds expectations, happiness is positive. But if our expectations or perceptions consistently extend beyond the reality of the situation, we are unhappy.

I'm not going to start telling you to lower expectations, as I think expecting more of yourself and more of your Hero's Journey is important. Instead, I just want you to be aware of that equation. Don't complain about what you don't have, and focus instead on what you DO have or on what you have accomplished.

As author and blogger Eric Barker points out on his site, Barking Up the Wrong Tree (bakadesuyo.com): "Bronze medalists are happier than silver medalists. This is because they feel grateful to get a medal at all. Silver medalists are left wondering what more they could have done to win, and bronze medalists are excited to be on the podium!"

So, in your quest for a leveled-up life, don't forget to also be grateful and thankful for the fact that your heart is still beating, that you have important people in your life who care about you, and you are working on leveling up. Consider this: When was the last time you handwrote a "thank-you" note? And how did you feel when you received one? Gratitude can go a long way and should be practiced as often as possible—it's a great way to stay present and grounded.

If you're interested in building the habit of gratitude, try writing down three things that went well every night before going to bed. Use Evernote, a Word doc, or a journal on your nightstand, but keep a record! Look back at the journal when you are feeling unhappy, and reflect on all the awesome things that have happened in your life recently. Don't finish one journey or mission and immediately move on to the next one. Instead, spend at least a few minutes enjoying the victory and being grateful for the opportunity.

FIND YOUR BALANCE

Just as there needs to be balance in the Force to bring peace to the Galaxy, we, too, need to have a balance in our lives that gives us the best chance to say, "Good game" on that game-over screen, whenever it may come. When somebody asks, "Did you enjoy your story?" I want you to say, "HELL YES." So how do we get there? In this nerd's humble opinion it's a combination of accomplishing goals, being present, and practicing gratitude that gives you the best chance to succeed in your journey toward a healthier body, a fulfilling career, and a life worth living.

I know this balance is important, which is why I make sure to devote at least a portion of every day to each of these things. I work hard to improve myself, but I also spend time reminding myself that, "Holy crap, I am alive! And that's amazing!" I remind myself that I'll never remember the work I did while skipping a friend's birthday party. We need to remember that life is meant to be lived, not endured.

Happiness is a consequence of the things you do daily, not a reward for earning a certain amount of money or purchasing a certain number of things. Find time every day to work on things that make you feel alive, with people that you love, and take a moment celebrate any victory, no matter how small—this will have you primed to rapidly advance in this Game of Life, and you'll have a blast along the way.

REBEL HERO

★ ★ ★ ★ ★ ★

NAME: Matt Storm   **AGE:** 30

HOMETOWN: Portland, OR

My job in clinical hematology allows me to encounter people on a daily basis nearing the end of their lives and taking a long, hard look back and seeing regret. You see that enough times and you realize you don't want to experience a lifetime of missed opportunities. I had allowed my circumstances to dictate my life, and I came to a point where I said enough was enough.

When I found Nerd Fitness it literally changed my life. I was never one to fit in with the crowd, but with Steve's help I've lost a cumulative 75 pounds and changed not only my body composition, but my outlook on life. Battling depression and dealing with the loss of a loved one to suicide led me to the Trevor Project where I am now a volunteer counselor. I talk with those who are going through tough times of

SPOTLIGHT

DAY JOB: *Bone Marrow and Stem Cell Transplant Coordinator*

ALTER EGO: *The Huntsman*   **CLASS:** *Assassin*

their own. I have a unique perspective with my day job, and I use my training to help guide youth. I try to be a beacon to them and help them to see another path out of their own darkness.

At the end of the day I'm able to head home where I'm fortunate enough to live next to a forest. There, I'm able to let out my inner assassin. Through parkour, gymnastics, and Primal Flow, I soar through the woods and release the pent-up emotions that are in my body and feel the adrenaline pump through my veins.

In addition to leveling up my life through physical activity and volunteering, I've also used my 20 seconds of courage to score another big victory: I just got the role of Roger in a local production of the musical *RENT!*

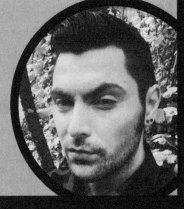

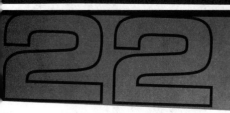

SHARE WHAT YOU'VE DISCOVERED AND LEARNED

The transformation and return of the hero is a critical component of his journey. This brings the story full circle and completes the quest. After the incident with the dragon, Bilbo returns to his home at Bag End and pens the events of the journey as: *The Hobbit: There and Back Again.* The "back again" part is crucial. We can't live out our entire existence as superheroes or spend all day every day in the supernatural world. It's important for us to return to the real world—whether it's returning to our day jobs after a week-long camping trip with our family, a return to school after competing in a Brazilian jujitsu tournament, or even just returning home after an evening of practicing violin. To complete the arc of the hero's journey, we need to go home again.

It took six long years of trials and tribulations before I finally found the formula for success in building a healthy body. I was so proud of and emboldened by the accomplishment that I became eager to share what I had learned through the experience with those who were interested in avoiding my mistakes. That decision ultimately resulted in the creation of Nerd Fitness, and now I get to serve as a Jedi Master to hundreds of thousands of people every day.

I felt the same way after I returned from my around-the-world trip. Things that had bothered me before became back-burner concerns and afterthoughts. Sitting in traffic or dealing with a delayed flight no longer sent my blood pressure soaring, because exploring the globe and learning the importance of enjoying the moment gave me a chance to reconfigure how I perceived everyday challenges.

It also gave me a chance to start sharing my knowledge with others in an effort to help them live adventurously, too. I received emails from folks all over the world asking for advice on where to stay in certain countries, or the cheapest way to experience a particular adventure, or how to get started with training in a particular skill. I'd learned from others, and because I had benefitted greatly from those mentors I was (and am) happy to pass along my knowledge. This has brought purpose and excitement to my life in a way that I'd never expected: I actually get more excited now about helping others accomplish a goal than I do from completing a goal myself. I can only imagine this is what a proud parent feels like when a child succeeds at something.

I want the same for you, and I believe you owe it to the world to share what you've learned. As you complete missions and quests and level up your life, you will transform: physically, mentally, and spiritually. Perhaps you lost a dramatic amount of weight, or completed a volunteering mission that put life into perspective, or you finally learned a skill that had eluded you for years. Whatever it is, when you cross an item off your quest list and return to the normal world, you'll actually start to live a dual existence. On one path, you are the hero who's following a Hero's Journey. On the other path, you become the mentor helping others along their own paths.

And that mentorship is important, because it actually becomes a different way for you to level up. As I said earlier in the book, when you teach somebody something, your knowledge of that subject can increase. As you get smarter and better at communicating the message, the more people you can help, and the better your advice becomes.

Alas, I need to share with you a word of warning: Only help those who ask for it. First, I spent months telling anybody who would listen how I got in shape and, later, I spent a few more months telling everyone about the new perspective I'd gained during my trip. Eventually, though, I came to a realization. When you emerge a changed hero after completing a quest in your Game of Life, you're faced with two choices: Do you come back and brag about the adventures you had? Or do you quietly go about your day knowing that few would ever understand what you just went through?

Although I love telling anybody who asks about my adventures, and I enjoy providing advice to people in the gym who ask about training in a particular exercise, I understand that telling everybody else what they're missing out on is a surefire way to get socked in the mouth. Nobody likes a know-it-all, and nobody likes to be told they are missing out because they haven't done something you've already done. On top of that, telling somebody who hasn't asked how to live their lives, or what they should be doing, is a great way to get them to do the exact opposite (sharing this book with your friends is totally okay though)!

Remember, we all have to start somewhere, and refusing the call of adventure is an important part of the story: Everybody has to find their own call to adventure—at their own pace—and to make the crucial decision to cross the threshold and take a chance when they are ready. If they don't make that decision, they're much more likely to give up at the first challenge along the way because their hearts were never in it.

I receive emails daily from concerned individuals asking me to motivate their loved ones to get in shape. "I'm getting healthy and improving," the emails say, "but I just can't get my husband/girlfriend/brother/friend to do the same. Help!" Unfortunately, as much as we would like to shake our friends and scream, "Wake up! You're burning daylight! Take control and get started!" It doesn't quite work that way. Remember, we were among the misinformed at one point, too, and it wasn't until we took control of our own destiny that we actually started to level up.

Instead, we need to do our best to channel our inner Captain America and inspire others through our actions. We can live our lives to the best of our ability and hopefully set the right kind of example. Others will be watching and taking notice, but only when they come to us asking for advice can we become a mentor to them. We can prepare to provide them with the tools they need to succeed, but they are the ones who have to pull the sword from the stone; they are the ones who have to take the red pill.

I would love for you to become a mentor in The Rebellion. We have a few hundred thousand members who are ready, willing, and able to take advice from those who have leveled up in the skills they wish to learn, or to visit places where they have already been.

Head on over to LevelUpYourLife.com and share your stories, struggles, adventures, and misadventures. I guarantee that no matter how small your victory, or how "normal" your quest might seem, there's somebody in The Rebellion who would love to hear about it and learn from you.

REBEL HERO

★ ★ ★ ★ ★ ★

NAME: Carrie McCrudden, MD   **AGE:** 44

HOMETOWN: Denver, CO

I am more of a bookworm than a gamer, but the level up concept has become totally central to my whole life approach. The whole idea of playing big instead of small, and peppering life with progressively larger adventures has characterized several years of massive change for me!

I have very well developed nerd credentials. I was the goofy kid in the corner with a book; uncoordinated, gangly, and severely poor at any team sport. My mom and my best friend's mom actually staged an intervention, due to an overall sense of panic at how much we were reading (a playdate for us back then consisted of reading encyclopedias . . . we spent our time comparing notes about which was better: Britannica or World), and refused to let me or my fabulous nerd partner in crime read until we had been outside for at least an hour. Naturally, we just brought our books outside. Eventually, I used my fabulous nerdiness to become a doctor and have happily been practicing as a psychologist specializing in helping teens and adults overcome trauma and learn to love their lives.

Along the way, it became apparent that I actually did like being physical, and I loved riding horses, hiking, and biking, but I never gave myself any credit since I didn't consider them "real sports." However, I liked being active and enjoyed being in shape. Around age 39, I started feeling frumpy and began

SPOTLIGHT

DAY JOB: *Psychologist*

ALTER EGO: *Doctor Carrie*   **CLASS:** *Warrior*

working out with a trainer. I set the goal of getting into the best shape of my life for my 40's. I began lifting, and lifting heavy, and eventually got convinced to enter into a powerlifting competition. Who knew it would be so fun? And I won! Huge surprise! Then, I competed in the Colorado state powerlifting competition, and set three state records. I have been competing ever since, and even got to compete at Nationals!

Along the way, I have decided to permanently level up my story about myself from bookish nerd in a corner to athletic, powerful nerd who is not hiding anymore! Now, I seek out the stuff I used to fear, or to think was good for others, but beyond my abilities. I've done silly, easy stuff like riding a mechanical bull. I've finally allowed myself to do things I wanted to try forever, like paragliding and Samba lessons. And, most of all, I have done huge things like believe in love again after a painful divorce. All along the way, getting fit, staying strong, and leveling up my stories about myself have been the central supports for this major change in my vision of myself.

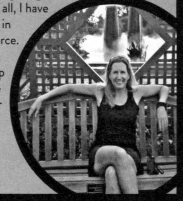

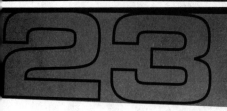

CONTINUE PLAYING FOR THE LOVE OF THE GAME

I leave you with a final parable: "The Tale of the Dragon Slayer."

The creature that fueled every decision you've made over the past few years is now a trophy mounted above your fireplace. The hours and days and weeks and months of blood, sweat, and tears resulted in an ultimate epic victory—something you never thought you'd achieve. *Life is different for you now.* You have a sense of accomplishment that you didn't know existed. The local townsfolk look at you differently as well: Tavern-dwellers are always eager to buy you a beer and hear the tale retold; even your old friends have a greater level of respect for you. All the children in town look up to you, pretending to slay their own dragons while running around the schoolyard.

And for a few weeks, life is grand.

The dragon has been slain, the day has been saved, and yet somehow something is missing. This tiny voice in the back of your mind tells you that your work isn't done. Sure, you can sit around for the rest of your life, getting fat and happy, reliving the glory days of that time you killed the dragon, and nobody would fault you—completing a major quest is nothing to scoff at. However, as the days go on, you start to realize more and more just how much the training you went through to fight that dragon meant—each day was filled with purpose, each step moving you one closer to a final battle.

With no dragon to fight, no mountain to climb, no treasure to discover, there's no real need to train with conviction anymore. Waking up early to work on sword skills or staying up late to practice archery no longer serve a purpose. Because nothing feels like a life-or-death situation, missed workouts or skill sessions are no longer a cause for concern. Pretty good is good enough. Mostly right is plenty. Tomorrow is a better day than today.

You've come to a crossroads, and you have a critical decision to make.

There are dragons and quests in all our lives. Some are big, some are small. Some are pushovers, and some require a few days of training to conquer, while others require an entire lifetime of dedication. These dragons are tough but not invincible, and one day they will fall. That's when the real work starts.

I ask you, my friend, what kind of dragon slayer will you be? Has-beens look back at what they've accomplished, pat themselves on the back, and give up doing everything that made them successful in the first place. The task is done, the item crossed off the list, and a "well-deserved break" quickly becomes permanent retirement. Nobody writes fairy tales about has-beens.

True dragon slayers stay hungry. After slaying a dragon and saving a town, they set their sights on a bigger dragon, on a bigger mountain, in a land even farther away. They understand that there's as much purpose in training for a quest as there is in completing it. They know that facing and defeating stronger adversaries will elevate them to an even-higher level. They don't say: "I can't wait 'til this is over," but rather, "I can't wait to find out what's next." *These are the slayers who live on in legends. These are the slayers who change history.*

Has-beens sit around talking about the dragon they slew. Real heroes find another dragon to slay! The world needs you to be a real hero.

THERE AND BACK AGAIN . . . AGAIN

The Hero's Journey is presented as a circle for one main reason: The sequence must repeat itself. The quest is never the same each time, and the stakes, enemies, and treasures are changing every time as well, but the hero must continually reinvent himself. Our Game of Life is not ONE big quest, but rather a series of smaller quests that all tie together, each time furthering the plot and advancing the development of our heroic arc. When you complete a major quest and return home, do take a few moments to celebrate with friends and family, or simply celebrate alone with your thoughts. If there's a chance to capture a memento or stick your achievement on the wall, go for it. You've earned it, and you should be proud of your accomplishments.

However, after a little while it's time to grab the sword, don your cape once again, and set out on another adventure. If your life is a movie, then you just got green-lit for a sequel with an even bigger budget. Maybe even more explosions. As Tom Hardy's character says in Christopher Nolan's *Inception:* "You mustn't be afraid to dream a little bigger, darling." Just don't forget the heart of what made the first story so successful: the development of your character, the embrace of your adventurous spirit, and the triumph over mediocrity, complacency, and boredom.

Your next quest awaits, adventurer, and we can't wait to see where it takes you.

DID YOU ENJOY YOUR STORY?

And thus we come to the conclusion, and I want to share with you one final thought. Although we don't get to pick how much time we have on this planet, there are two things we do get to control:

1. Who we spend our time with.
2. The memories we collect with those people.

Want a recipe for success and happiness? Spend as much time as you can with the people you love, and put yourself in as many situations as possible with those people who enable you to look back and say, "Man, remember that time we . . . ; I can't believe that actually happened!"

There are many things people take for granted, but none more so than our health and the time we might have left. We can directly control one, and we have minimal control over the other, so we might as well enjoy today, right? Every day is an opportunity to level up, to improve, to learn, and to grow. This is an opportunity that so many people who have passed away would have given anything to regain: the chance to live adventurously in whatever manner you see fit, with the people who mean the most to you. I'm going to leave you with a final quote from *The Shawshank Redemption*:

> I FIND I'M SO EXCITED I CAN HARDLY SIT STILL OR HOLD A THOUGHT IN MY HEAD. I THINK THAT'S SOMETHING ONLY A FREE MAN CAN FEEL—A FREE MAN AT THE START OF A LONG JOURNEY WHOSE CONCLUSION IS UNCERTAIN.

I'm excited to follow along with your adventure over at LevelUpYourLife.com, and watch how you've chosen to play the Game of Life. I can't wait to see what kind of hero you'll become. Whether it's learning a new language or traveling the globe, building a school in Africa or taking your kids on a weekend hiking trip, adventure is out there. Not only that, but now you have all of the tools and information you need to get started. And that's all that's left: to get started. Today.

Good luck, and I'll see you at the top of the mountain!

RESOURCES OF THE REBELLION

Want to know the secret to getting ahead and continuing to level up every single day? There are two key things that I've noticed nearly every successful person I admire does on a regular basis: They exercise, and they read voraciously. They're never without a book or Kindle, learning about the next big thing, planning their personal development, or discovering ways how to improve themselves. Whether smart people read, or reading makes people smarter is up for debate—I would argue it's both! Here's why I read up to two books a week:

1. I read fiction books at night while in bed to help me fall asleep. Instead of staring at a TV that makes me anxious, or a computer/TV screen while gaming, I'm in bed reading about Middle Earth, or Hogwarts, the people of Hugh Howey's Silo trilogy, or what predicament Jack Reacher has gotten himself into. This gives my brain a chance to shut down and not think about leveling up.

2. I read nonfiction books to help me in my business and in my life. Whether I'm reading books that help me build better systems to get more done in less time, books on happiness and how our brains are wired, or even books on certain countries

that inspire me to travel, reading helps me level up my life. I also LOVE reading books about how successful people got their start.

Now, we've already covered why "I don't have time" is not a good excuse anymore. If you don't have time to read, where are your priorities? I read on my Kindle while on a plane, while waiting in line at Chipotle, before I go to bed, when I wake up, while eating lunch, instead of watching TV, while sitting by the pool. I try to fill up my free time with reading. I encourage you to do the same. However, remember that reading can be the equivalent of collecting underpants; don't forget to take action!

Here, I present you with a list of my favorite resources. They include books on language learning or travel, inspirational movies that will encourage you me to get off your butt and find adventure, and websites that can help you develop new skills to change careers. You can find relevant links to access or purchase these resources at LevelUpYourLife.com.

HEALTH AND FITNESS

NerdFitness.com: I bet you saw that coming, right? Ha! Two free articles every week, a massive community full of supportive Rebels from all over the world, and some elite resources for people who want more specific advice on a wide variety of topics. Start here and check the resources I recommend through the site!

TRAVEL RESOURCES

NomadicMatt.com: One of the premier travel websites out there, especially if you are interested in traveling on a budget or interested in long-term travel.

LegalNomads.com: Jodi Etternberg is a lawyer turned full-time traveler. If you are a solo female traveler, this site is a must read!

ThePointsGuy.com: Interested in travel hacking? Look no further than ThePointsGuy.com, whose daily emails really help teach you which cards or offers will get you to the places you want to go. Most helpful for U.S. citizens.

LevelUpYourLife.com: In addition to allowing you to build your own character, this site also houses my favorite resources for travel hacking, trip planning, and packing.

LANGUAGE LEARNING

FluentIn3Months.com: How to learn any language quickly; the site is run by Benny Lewis.

iTalki.com: Find virtual tutors via Skype in the language you want to learn.

DuoLingo.com: Gamify your language learning!

PERSONAL DEVELOPMENT AND BUSINESS BUILDING

FourHourWorkWeek.com: Run by Tim Ferrris, a fantastic blog on life hacking, personal development, travel, physical excellence, and more.

ChrisGuillebeau.com: I'm proud to call Chris a friend and mentor. It was his free ebook *279 Days to Overnight Success* that gave me a path to follow for my own site.

IWillTeachYouToBeRich.com: Run by Ramit Sethi, this site helped me get my financial life together, teaching me how to automate finances and more.

Fizzle.co: If you are interested in building a small online business, this is my favorite resource. Chase and Corbett are friends and two of the good guys in the often sketchy world of online business.

LiveYourLegend.net: Run by the late Scott Dinsmore, a great dude whose TEDx talk has been seen by over a million people. Scott helps people find their passion and live life deliberately.

Nerdist.com: Created by Chris Hardwick, king of the nerds. Think of this like a one-stop shop for all of your nerdy news needs.

WRITING A BOOK

GoinsWriter.com: Jeff Goins lives in Nashville and helps people discover their passion for writing, encouraging people to travel and find their calling.

Scrivener: I used this software to write this book. The program allows you to set daily goals and gamify your writing process!

LEARNING NEW SKILLS

KhanAcademy.com: Interested in math? Science? Ancient history? Learn from professionals. For free. Never stop learning!

Code Academy: If you are interested in learning a new programming language, you might as well start today. Free and interactive, Code Academy is a great way to begin your coding adventure.

TED.com: Inspirational 15-minute talks from some of the world's thought leaders. Impossible to not get inspired.

BOOKS I LOVE

The 4-Hour Workweek, by Tim Ferriss. I bought this book on a lunch break, read it in a day, and bought NerdFitness.com just a few days later. This is the go-to resource for lifestyle design, and the book that changed everything for me.

How to Travel the World on $50 a Day, by Matt Kepnes. Creator of NomadicMatt.com, Matt dispels the myth that travel needs to be expensive.

Losing My Virginity, by Richard Branson. The book that drastically altered what I thought I could accomplish with my own business. Reads like an adventure novel!

The Nerdist Way, by Chris Hardwick. A fantastic book on personal development that helps nerds make sense of life. If you're a fan of Chris's work or just a fan of nerd culture in general, go for it.

I Will Teach You To Be Rich, by Ramit Sethi. A must read for anybody trying to get their financial situation together. This book seriously changed my financial health and should be recommended reading for everybody.

The Alchemist, by Paulo Coelho. A fictional story that is full of parables and lessons about going on a journey. I read this book at least once a year.

The Writer's Journey, by Christopher Vogler. How the Hero's Journey applies to some of the most popular movies out there, including the Star Wars series.

Ready Player One, by Ernest Cline. A fictional story, but if you happen to be a child of the '80s or love pop culture, this is a no-brainer. I read it in a single sitting.

MOVIES I LOVE

The Shawshank Redemption. This movie has changed my life, and it inspired a mission on my Epic Quest of Awesome. Guaranteed to give me tears by the end. If you haven't seen it, drop what you're doing and watch it. Now.

The Secret Life of Walter Mitty (2013). Great soundtrack, and everybody can relate to Walter, a normal Joe with a regular job who decides to start living. I found myself cheering by the end of it.

Captain America: The First Avenger. My favorite superhero's origin story. Doesn't get much better than this.

The Goonies. A group of kids in a sleepy town find a treasure map and go on an adventure in their own backyard. Pirates! Mobsters! Gold! What's not to love?

Star Wars IV: A New Hope. Hopefully this goes without saying, but this is the movie that started it all for many of us nerds. Even if you've seen it a million times, it might be a good time to return to the Star Wars universe.

The Bourne Identity. Watch this and tell me you don't want to travel the world, have Swiss bank accounts, speak multiple languages, learn martial arts, and disappear at the drop of a hat; I dare you.

JOIN THE REBELLION

I n 2009, I started a fitness blog that provided health and fitness tips encouraging nerds to get started living healthier lives. That site is NerdFitness.com, and it has since evolved into something far greater than I ever could have imagined. What was once a blog is now a worldwide movement of Rebels from nearly every country who are working hard to live better lives. We are a ragtag bunch of misfits that level up our lives every single day, and we would love to help you on your own journey to a better life.

Whether you're looking to lose weight, build muscle, or simply start living a life that makes you proud, join us. Receive free weekly emails full of education and inspiration, and participate in a thriving community that offers support and guidance. Track your own epic quest and share stories with others.

You can even create your own character for free, complete missions and quests, and level up your character as you get in shape. If you are interested in more advanced information, with training videos, worksheets, and expert knowledge in the subjects that matter to you, then check it out.

In addition to a supportive online community, we also host in-person events throughout the year that will give you a chance to connect with fellow Rebels in your area or to learn from members of Team Nerd Fitness on a wide variety of topics. Every year we host events like Camp Nerd Fitness, where Rebels can spend a long weekend with each other learning new skills in a safe environment and have a damn good time doing it.

Remember, we don't care where you came from, only where you're going! See you in the community!

LevelUpYourLife.com

ACKNOWLEDGMENTS

First, a massive thanks to the members of The Rebellion at Nerd Fitness. What started as a boy and his blog is now a diverse community of people I'm proud to call my friends. Thank you for taking action, leveling up your lives, and inspiring me to get better every day. Never stop pushing and never stop growing. Also, thanks to the other members of Team Nerd Fitness for giving me the opportunity to take a chance on writing a book, and for putting up with my crazy ideas. Let's make our dent in the universe.

Next, thanks to the wonderful wizards over at Rodale, specifically my editor, Mark Weinstein, who helped me lift this literary X-wing out of the swamp and back into flight. To my friend Matt Gartland, thanks for taking this chaotic mess of movie references and video game metaphors and turning it into something that can help others. I'm not sure how we pulled it off, but here we are. Thanks to my agent David Fugate, who patiently put up with me for years before I finally worked up the courage to write *Level Up Your Life.*

I want to also thank some of my heroes: Tim Ferriss, whose book, *The 4-Hour Workweek,* inspired me to start Nerd Fitness just days after reading it. To Chris Guillebeau, who has served as my Yoda and mentor throughout nearly my entire journey. To Brett McKay, who taught me how powerful a great community can be and who helped me find my footing when I was just starting out.

To Chris Hardwick, thanks for replying to one of my emails when I first started my site—I never forgot it. To Andy Levine, my former boss at Sixthman, thanks for being the "best man I ever worked for," and showing me how to build a community and company right. To Adam Baker, thanks for teaching me how to NOT suck at blogging. To Staci Ardison, thanks for taking a chance and helping me to build Nerd Fitness into what it is today—we're just getting started! To Marco (aka PM), thanks for your fantastic mixes—they've gotten me through hundreds of hours of content creation.

Thanks to Shigeru Miyamoto, for teaching me that a small boy with pointy ears and a wooden sword can change the fate of Hyrule. Thanks to Richard Branson, who inspired me to think big but never lose sight of the true purpose: to be happy and do good. Thanks to J.R.R. Tolkien, who taught me that "not all those who wander are lost," and to Stan Lee, for creating the wonderful Marvel universe that keeps us nerds excited and inspired.

I would also like to thank Captain America, who taught me to stick to my values when the easier path lay elsewhere; Frodo, who taught me that the only way to get to Mordor is one step at a time; Yoda, who reminded me to "do or do not, there is no try"; Harry Potter, who gave every kid a chance to dream that they could be a wizard; Jason Bourne, who taught me how to be resilient and calm under pressure, no matter where in the world I was; and James Bond, who taught me witty catchphrases, and that tuxes never go out of style.

Thanks to my Grampy, who taught me to live a life worth living but to never take things too seriously; to Nana, who taught me "of course you can," and to my Grampa, who inspired me to volunteer, never complain, and take action. I miss you all terribly, and I'm lucky that I got a chance to grow up knowing you.

A huge shout out to my goofball friends: Cash McLaughlin, thanks for convincing me to go on crazy trips. Chris St. James, thanks for being there daily to listen to my crazy ideas. Eric Hannah, thanks for helping kickstart my entrepreneurial spirit with our thriving friendship bracelet business in 3rd grade (I still owe you $20). Joe Rougeux, I couldn't be more proud of you man—congrats on leveling up with Hi-Rez Studios. Adam Moore and Tyler Thompson, for inviting me to mogul lunches in Nashville. Oh, and Greg Lamas . . . don't ever change.

Lastly, thanks again to my family. Jack, thanks for being a good big brother and for giving me somebody to look up to since day one. Emily, thanks for always being so damn excited to hang out with me—your positive attitude is infectious, keep it up! Gramma, thanks for being such a big fan of my work, even though you don't get most of the references! Finally, to Mom and Dad. Thanks for never doubting me, always supporting me, and being my biggest fans and marketers. I love you.

INDEX

Boldface page references indicate photographs and illustrations. <u>Underscored</u> references indicate boxed text.

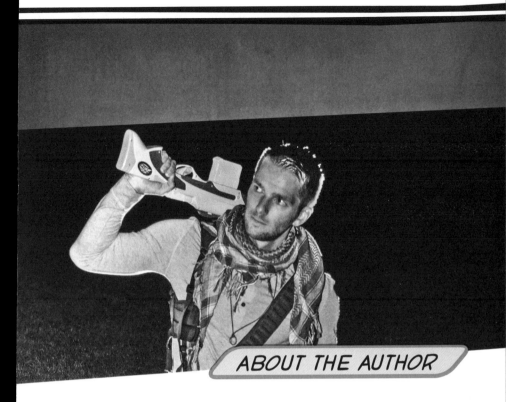

Many people believe that Steve Kamb was created in a laboratory in the 1940s as part of a top-secret government program to fight the Nazis. Those people are wrong; that was Steve Rogers, and he became Captain America. But close enough.

Steve Kamb was born on Cape Cod, Massachusetts, raised by two loving parents and a Nintendo Entertainment System. When he wasn't getting lost in video games, he spent his childhood playing tennis baseball in the streets, building tree forts in the backyard, and participating in neighborhood-wide games of capture the flag.

Upon graduating from Vanderbilt University in 2006, he began developing the idea for a website to help beginners get healthy and avoid all of the usual pitfalls. Years later, that site became NerdFitness.com, a now-worldwide fitness community dedicated to helping nerds, desk jockeys, and self-aware robots level up their lives.

While running his company from a coconut laptop, Steve has adventured all over the world, explored the ruins of Machu Picchu, dived with sharks on the Great Barrier Reef, and lived like James Bond in Monte Carlo. He has guest lectured at Google, Google Dublin, Facebook, TEDxEmory, and regularly speaks at Vanderbilt University.

He recently moved from Nashville, Tennessee, to New York City to continue his quest of becoming Captain America. He spends his free time picking up heavy things, singing off-key, and playing music as loudly as possible. He hopes to one day own an island in the Caribbean, be part of a heist, and reach level 50 in the Game of Life.

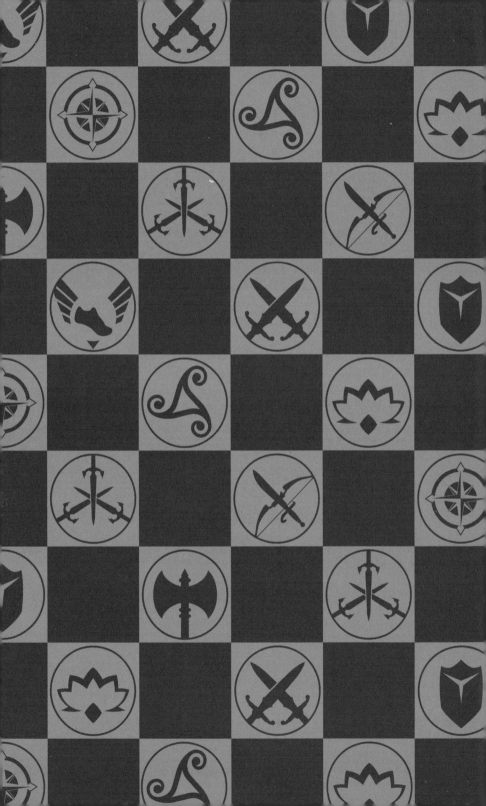